Inpatient Obstetric Nurse Exam Study Guide

RNC- OB Exam Review Book

with Practice Questions and Rationale

Sandra H. White
© 2023-2024
Printed in USA.

Disclaimer

Contents

Clear the Inpatient Obstetric Nurse® Exam easily using the Success Secrets in this book!

What are the Secrets?

• Frequently Asked Questions: Questions are prepared based on the latest curriculum. The frequently asked questions are given to make you familiarize with the important concepts.

• Sharpen your thinking ability: Our explanation to the practice question will help you to improve your reasoning ability and hence you will be able to answer any type of question with ease.

• Repeated mind training: The more you train your mind to read and understand different types questions and answers, it becomes easier to answer any type of question in the RNC-OB ® exam . There are 300+ questions in this book to give you a clear idea of all the concepts covered in the exam.

• No last minute surprise: These questions and options are designed in a way that matches the Inpatient Obstetric Nurse Exam so that you don't have a feeling of embarrassment when you take the actual exam.

• More weightage, more exploration: Certain concepts like **Labor and Birth (35%), Complications of Pregnancy (29%)** and **Fetal Assessment (18%)** are given more weightage in the Inpatient Obstetric Nurse ®Exam. Hence we have covered more around these topics which will help you to dive deep in the core concepts and easily pass the exam.

Why this book?

• All the question in this book are prepared and reviewed by Experts considering the latest curriculum.

• The question and option format exactly matches the actual Inpatient Obstetric Nurse Exam so that the test takers will get an idea and experience of attending the exam.

• There are 3000+ RNC-OB® Exam Practice Questions so that you are clear with all the concepts and gain 100% confidence before taking the RNC Exam.

• For every question there is an explanation for the correct answer which will make you to understand the concepts clearly, in case if you are not sure of.

• The questions in this book are prepared on the basis of the following Inpatient Obstetric Nurse Exam content outline :

Domain I: Complications of Pregnancy (29%)

Domain II: Fetal Assessment (18%)

Domain III: Labor and Birth (35%)

Domain IV: Recovery, Postpartum and Newborn Care (15%)

Domain V: Professional Issues(3%)

• More Weightage, More Number of Questions for that concept. The questions are randomly ordered just as in the actual RNC-OB exam to improve thinking ability.

Wishing you all the best! You will be a proud Inpatient Obstetric Nurse soon!

Inpatient Obstetric Nurse Exam Practice Questions

Question 1:   Which of the laws listed below enables people with disabilities to accommodate in doctor's offices?
A) Health insurance act
B) Disability privilege act
C) Americans with disabilities act (ADA)
D) Disabilities insurance act

Question 2:   Which of the following is not a sign of ectopic pregnancy?
A. Pain in the abdomen
B. Vaginal bleeding.
C. Aversion to certain foods
D. None of the above.

Question 3:   Which among the following is true about preeclampsia?
A.   It is a multisystem disorder
B.   It is commonly seen as associated with maternal hypertension
C.   Swelling in the legs and increased water retention
D.   All of the above

Question 4:   Which of the following will rightly define Placenta Previa?
A. Infection in the uterus.
B.   Endocervical os with placenta overlaying.
C. Fetal vessel rupture
D. Infection in the placenta.

Question 5:   On auscultation of the fetal heart rate it is found to be 140 beats per minute which is considered to be normal. What range of fetal heart rate is considered to be normal?
A.   110 to 140 beats per minute
B.   110 to 160 beats per minute
C.   120 to 140 beats per minute
D.   130 to 200 beats per minute

Question 6:   A 28-week pregnant lady came to the department of gynecology with symptoms suggestive of bacterial vaginosis. Among the following, all are suggestive of bacterial vaginosis except _____.

A.   Pyrexia and symptoms suggestive of flu
B.   Burning Urination
C.   Fishy odor in discharge
D.   Vaginal discharge that is grey or white

Question 7:   Melissa a 28-year-old female is in her 38th week of pregnancy. She has come to the OPD for the following symptoms: fatigue, nausea, swelling of the extremities, and breathlessness. Lab diagnosis reveals proteinuria. What is the most probable diagnosis?

A.   Hyperglycemia
B.   Epilepsy
C.   Preeclampsia
D.   Renal failure correct

Question 8:   In which of the following condition is Magnesium sulfate prescribed between **24 and 36 weeks**?

A. Increase the lung maturity of the baby.
B. To reduce the risk of brain damage to the baby.
C. To avoid pre-term labor.
D. Both B and C

Question 9:   A patient with 38 weeks of gestation is showing symptoms of hypovolemia. On monitoring the fetal heart rate it is noted that there is fetal bradycardia . What is the most probable diagnosis?

A.   Uterine Rupture
B.   Esophageal malformation
C.   Rh incompatibility
D.   None of the above

Question 10:   International Society of thrombosis and hemostasis course range from_____.

A.   0-9
B.   0-8
C.   2-8
D.   3-16

Question 11: A woman who is 40 weeks into gestation is yet to deliver the fetus has opted for an elective C-section. She is having prolonged labor. Prior to the procedure, she is administered Oxytocin. Which among the following are the functions of Oxytocin?
A. Induces labor
B. Lowers postpartum blood loss by controlling hemorrhage
C. Reducing anxiety
D. All of the above

Question 12: A medical practice that violates ethical or legal standards or is irresponsible and illegal is_____:
A. Malpractice.
B. Reporting Choice
C. Flexible reimbursement.
D. Effective practice

Question 13: Which of the following is the grating or crackling in the ribs of a newborn?
A. Rib fracture
B. Murmur
C. Crepitus.
D. Hardley's response.

Question 14: Which of the following does not cause placental insufficiency?
A. Surgery.
B. Diabetes Mellitus.
C. Hypothyroidism.
D. Anemia.

Question 15: Sodium ferric gluconate is being given via IV infusion to a pregnant woman. Which dose among the following is to be chosen?
A. 135 mg given in 1000 ml normal saline
B. 150 mg given in 100 ml ringer lactate
C. 125 mg given in 100 ml ringer's lactate
D. 125 mg given in 100ml normal saline

Question 16: To evaluate the physical health of the mother and fetus all except which of the following are to be included?
A. Fetal movement
B. Uterine activity
C. Fetal heart rate

D.   Socio-economic status of the family

Question 17:   Donna is a known case of scleroderma. She is planning to get pregnant. Which type of scleroderma is safe so that pregnancy will not be a problem?
A) Systemic
B) Localized
C) Mutant
D) Variable

Question 18:   Dorsiflexion or Homans' sign indicate?
A.   Deep vein thrombosis (DVT).
B.   Swelling
C.   Purpura.
D.   Inflammation.

Question 19:   Which of the following might cause fetal bradycardia?
A. Maternal Pneumonia
B. Fetal palpitations.
C. Umbilical cord compression for a long time
D. Polyploidy

Question 20:   Prior to cleaning the mucus from an infant's nose and mouth. What should the nurse do first?
A.   Remove the mucus from the nose and mouth using suction.
B.   Place the tip directly in the back of the infant's mouth.
C.   Gently place the tip of the bulb in the infant's nose.
D.   Prior to placing the syringe tip into the infant's mouth, depress the bulb.

Question 21:   Which of the following is not the symptom of a UTI (urinary tract infection)?
A. Burning sensation and pain during urination
B. Cloudy urine.
C. Foul-smelling urine.
D. Shortness of breath.

Question 22: A baby born 4 days ago is being breastfed. What should be the color of the stool of the new born on the 5th day?

A.   Bright yellow.

B.   Brown.

C.   Black.

D.   Green.

Question 23: Which of the following level of amniotic fluid is described as the condition of polyhydramnios?

A. More than 8 cm maximum pool.

B. Less than 8 cm maximum pool.

C. AFI less than 38 cm.

D. 6000 ml of amniotic fluid.

Question 24: Cheryl has delivered a baby. She is a non-lactating mother. How long will it take for her to resume her periods?

A) 4-6 weeks

B) 7-9 weeks

C) 12-16weeks

D) >16 weeks

Question 25: Choose the terms from the following options that describe the premature separation of a normal implanted placenta.

A. Miscarriage

B. Placental abruption.

C. Ovarian cyst

D. Molar pregnancy

Question 26: Which among these is a cause of an infant being unable to pass meconium?

A.   Meconium plug syndrome

B.   Dehydration

C.   Already passed meconium in the uterus

D.   Both B and C

Question 27: How does pregnancy affect the abdominal wall?

A.   The abdominal wall is weakened and muscle tone is diminished.

B.   The abdominal wall is strengthened.

C.   The abdominal wall becomes resilient to pain.

D. Muscle tone becomes easier to shape and form.

Question 28: During the newborn screening process in the U.S., all babies are tested for _____ metabolic disorder.

A. Phenylketonuria
B. Alexander disease.
C. Prader Willi syndrome.
D. Color blindness.

Question 29: A neonate showing symptoms of neonatal abstinence syndrome such as seizures and tremors is to be treated by which of the following?

A. Swaddling the infant tightly
B. Placing the infant in sunlight
C. Placing the infant in skin-to-skin contact
D. Both A and C

Question 30: A pregnant woman is diagnosed with polyhydramnios. What does this diagnosis mean?

A. It is an excess of amniotic fluid seen mostly during the second trimester of pregnancy
B. It is the deficiency of amniotic fluid
C. It is excessive loss of amniotic fluid
D. It is a sudden rupture of the placenta

Question 31: Wharton's Jelly supplies blood to placenta. Wharton's Jelly envelops the umbilical cord, provides cushioning effect, and protects the umbilical cord. Which of the following is true when the blood vessels in the umbilical cord do not have Wharton's jelly to protect them and cross the membranes before joining to form the chord?

A. Causes protracted labor
B. Placenta Previa
C. Abruptio placenta
D. Velamentous cord insertion

Question 32: If a woman has depression during her pregnancy the infant is most likely to have all except which among the following:

A. Asthma

B.   Underweight
C.   Premature birth
D.   Irritable infant

Question 33:   Which of the following is the right term to describe the condition when the cervix does not stay closed during pregnancy?
A. Cervical dissolution
B. Cervical incompetence.
C. Cervical myelopathy.
D. Cervical widening

Question 34: Hannah who is 14 weeks pregnant has previous history of migraine. During pregnancy, her symptoms of migraine are likely to _____.
A.   Worsen
B.   Remain constant
C.   Improve
D.   Develop complications

Question 35:   Maria a 28-year-old woman delivered an infant weighing 8 Pounds and 13 ounces which is more than the average weight. This condition is called fetal macrosomia. What is the most common cause associated with this condition?
A.   Diabetes mellitus
B.   Obesity
C.   Overdue pregnancy
D.   All of the above

Question 36:   A mother delivers an infant weighing 4 pounds and 8 ounces is said to have delivered preterm. Preterm is a condition where contractions occur how many weeks before the due date?
A.   40
B.   28
C.   37
D.   39

Question 37: Sharon complaints of golf ball-sized blood clots in her lochia. Which is NOT suspected in her?
A) Deep venous thrombosis (DVT)
B) Bleeding
C) Retained placental bits
D) Birth canal lacerations

Question 38: _____ cue of readiness is shown by the new born if the newborn is seeking and rooting with the opened mouth?
A. Late.
B. Mid.
C. Early.
D. Moderate.

Question 39: Which sleep state is a newborn in when he is startled awake by sudden noises, twitching his arms and legs, and moving his eyes rapidly beneath closed lids?
A.   Calm sleep
B.   Unwinded sleep
C.   Active sleep
D.   REM sleep

Question 40: A patient in the maternity ward has delivered a baby. To prevent a DVT (deep vein thrombosis) which of the following interventions by a nurse will NOT be favorable?
A. Complete bed rest.
B. Hydration.
C. Immediate ambulation.
D. All of the above.

Question 41: In order to suppress lactation, which medication is prescribed?
A.   Desvenlafaxine
B.   Zoloft
C.   Trazodone
D.   Estrogen.

Question 42: Patricia, a 28-year-old female in her second pregnancy, is found to be carrying a fetus that is Rh-positive. The mother is Rh negative. Following delivery, the baby shows signs of hemorrhagic disease of the newborn. It is caused due to?

A. Hepatic failure
B. Deficiency of vitamin K
C. Hypothermia
D. Hypoglycemia

Question 43: How is Cystic fibrosis from the mother passed on to the infant?

A. Genetically.
B. Birth canal infection.
C. Bloodstream of the mother.
D. Unknown factors.

Question 44: What would NOT be considered an intervention that might help a postpartum patient who has hemorrhoid discomfort?

A. Baths with sitz positions
B. Medicine applications
C. Antibiotics
D. The use of ice packs

Question 45: A patient has suffered a trauma and died. The patient is not pregnant. Which of the following will be considered the cause of death?

A. Epilepsy
B. Hemorrhage.
C. Hyperglycemia.
D. Cardiac arrest.

Question 46: Sarah who is pregnant had a separation of abdominal muscles. What is the condition called?

A) Ascites
B) Amoeboma
C) Diastasis recti abdominis
D) Lochia Alba

Question 47: While administering misoprostol for postpartum bleeding, which route would be considered correct?

A. Aurally
B. Rectally
C. Intramuscular

D.   IV

Question 48:   Sometimes there exists decelerations or accelerations in the fetal heart rate. It corresponds to uterine contractions which is known as which of the following?
A. Periodic changes.
B. Irregular heart rate.
C. FHR up and down
D. FHR AD

Question 49:   Involution is improved by all factors EXCEPT:
A.   Labor that is not complicated.
B.   Bottle feeding.
C.   Sooner ambulation.
D.   Expulsion of placenta and membranes to the fullest extent possible.

Question 50:   During child birth in which of the following options does the cervical tear happen?
A. Nausea
B. Low level placenta previa.
C. Severe morning sickness during pregnancy.
D. Overweight

Question 51:   Why are twins/triplets/quintuplets often born prematurely before the seventh month?
A) Due to space occupancy by the fetuses there is over distension of the uterus triggering early labor
B) There is decreased blood supply to the fetuses
C) There is hyper coagulation which triggers delivery
D) None of the above

Question 52:   Type of abruptio placenta that causes vaginal bleeding is_____?
A.   Marginal
B.   Partial
C.   Complete
D.   Both B and C

Question 53:   A 30-week pregnant woman shows cutaneous purpura, easy bruisability and blood clots which are suggestive of disseminated intravascular coagulation. All of the following predispose to disseminated intravascular coagulation EXCEPT :

A. Diabetes mellitus
B. Abruptive placenta
C. Sepsis
D. Preeclampsia

Question 54: **Which of the following will NOT be included in the symptoms of chlamydia?**
A. Irregular periods
B. Dizziness.
C. Abdominal pain.
D. Painful intercourse.

Question 55: **Toxoplasmosis caused by T.gondii is transmitted by all of the following EXCEPT?**
A. Cat feces
B. Undercooked meat
C. Unused blood
D. Over cooked meat causing denaturation of muscle

Question 56: **Choose the correct option. What is the ideal time or frequency for checking the vital signs post-delivery when the patient is in the postpartum state after a normal delivery?**
A. Every 30 minutes for 3 hours.
B. Every 10 minutes for 30 minutes and then every 5 minutes for 24 hours.
C. Every 15 minutes for 1 hour and then every 30 minutes for 2 hours.
D. Every 4 hours.

Question 57: **Postpartum pain relief can be achieved with any of the following methods, EXCEPT for:**
A. Drugs that are mildly narcotic
B. The use of hot packs.
C. Getting a mas
D. Drugs that are heavily narcotic

Question 58: **A baby's skin creases appear to be especially notable for this rash, which can be reddish, raw, and very intense :**
A. Hives
B. psoriasis.
C. Tinea cruris.

D.   Intertrigo

Question 59:   A woman suffers nervous system damage during pregnancy or after birth. Which of the following conditions causes a loss in the ability to control muscles?
A. Meningocele
B. Cerebral Palsy.
C. Parkinsonism
D. Epilepsy

Question 60:   What is a trapped placenta?
A.   It is a lack of expulsion of placenta within 30 minutes of delivery of infant
B.   It is caused due to closure of the cervix before the placenta is expelled
C.   It increases the chances of postpartum hemorrhage
D.   All of the above

Question 61:   Ria a pregnant woman walked into the OPD and was diagnosed with cervical insufficiency. Which is NOT the symptom that may be seen?
A) Variable/ectopic pulse
B) Pressure symptoms of protrusion or something from the vagina
C) Bleeding from the vagina
D) Vaginal discharge

Question 62:   Choose the correct answer. Find out the abnormal score for an amniotic fluid index (AFI).
A. AFI =10 cm
B. AFI = 5 cm
C. AFI = 25 cm
D. AFI = 20 cm

Question 63:   In a fetus, which period is the most likely risk for developing gross abnormalities?
A. 2nd trimester.
B. 3rd trimester.
C. None.
D. 1st trimester.

Question 64:   Jenny 24-year-old woman 12 weeks into gestation is found to have carrying a fetus whose Rh positive, Jenny is Rh negative. The consequence of this would be _____ ?
A.   Breakdown of erythrocytes

B.   Breakdown of leukocytes
C.   Reduced immunity
D.   Impress immunoglobulin function

Question 65: **During 28 weeks of pregnancy fetal development mainly focuses on which among the following?**
A.   Development of focus to accommodate objects 8 to 12 inches away
B.   Growth and development of the fetus to survive in the external environment
C.   Development of fully functioning ears
D.   Development of hand and eye coordination

Question 66: **On ultrasound on a 28 year old pregnant women it was seen that there was excess amniotic fluid around the fetus. This condition is termed as?**
A.   Polyhydramnios
B.   Oligohydramnios
C.   Abnormal volume of fluid
D.   None of the above

Question 67: **At the time of labor through which among the following pathways does amniotic fluid enter maternal circulation?**
A.   Diffuses via placenta
B.   Via an umbilical cord
C.   Via point of separation of the placenta
D.   Both a and c

Question 68: **When does miscarriage, also called the spontaneous abortion occur?**
A. Before 20 weeks of pregnancy.
B. Before 22 weeks of pregnancy.
C. Before 25 weeks of pregnancy.
D. Before 30 weeks of pregnancy.

Question 69: **Kate , a 30-year-old patient is 33 weeks pregnant. She is admitted to the ER due to abdominal pain , shoulder pain, and vomiting. The BP was recorded to be 135/80 mm of hg and pulse 84 beats per minute. The fetal heart sounds were not heard. What is suspected in this case?**
A.   Hepatic Hematoma
B.   Hepatic rupture
C.   Hypovolemic shock
D.   None of the above

Question 70: Which of the following is NOT a key responsibility of the nurse at the latent stage of labor?
A. Watch for uterine atony.
B. Lamaze breathing to be taught to the mother.
C. Help with comfort and positioning.
D. Keep encouraging the mother and the partner.

Question 71: Dissipation of fetus's own created heat occurs through which of the following structures?
A) The mother's vagina
B) The fetal and placental membranes
C) Through the mother's umbilicus
D) There is no dissipation of heat

Question 72: As a response to physiology, what is the normal amount of body weight a newborn can afford to lose in the first 1 week of life?
A) 3-5%
B) 5-10%
C) 10-20%
D) 20-30%

Question 73: For a nurse who is examining a patient's lochia, _____ is NOT a factor to examine?
A) Clots
B) Weight
C) Odor
D) Color

Question 74: Which of the following reports the external electronic fetal monitoring?
A. Ultrasound is used to measure the fetal heart rate. Contractions are measured using a pressure sensor.
B. An electrode is used to measure the fetal heart rate. They are inserted into the vagina and cervix to reach the fetal scalp.
C. Manual examination is done using the two fingers against the fetal windpipe.
D. Fetal heart rate is measured using electrocardiography.

Question 75: Newborn mortality is primarily caused by which of the following factors?
A.   Cardiac arrest

B.   Pancytopenia
C.   Embolism
D.   Congenital abnormalities

Question 76:   Fetal kick count is evaluated in a woman who is 34 weeks pregnant. Among the following which one is considered to be the prime necessity for performing fetal kick count evaluation?
A.   To measure the fetal well-being and fetal oxygen supply
B.   To measures the fetal growth
C.   To measures the fetal hemoglobin level
D.   To measure the contraction rate

Question 77:   Stacy was blessed with a baby boy who became pale and had difficulty breathing when he attained the age of one month. What could be the cause of this?
A) The child suffered from Rh incompatibility
B) The child may have a history of birth trauma
C) His bone marrow does not produce enough blood cells
D) All of the above

Question 78:   The inability of newborns to regulate heat presents with a skin condition called?
A) Seborrhoea
B) Scabies
C) Miliria (prickly heat)
D) Angioedema

Question 79:   The number of phases seen in amniotic fluid embolism is?
A.   2
B.   4
C.   3
D.   6

Question 80:   On an average what is the normal rate of respiration seen in a newborn?
A) 10-20 cycles per minute
B) 20-40 cycles per minute
C) 40-60 cycles per minute
D) 60-100 cycles per minute

Question 81:   Shirley is a premature baby born with respiratory distress. The reason was found to be apnea. What is the anatomical cause of apnea?

A) Inadequate amounts of surfactant production
B) Diaphragmatic malfunction and development
C) Atelectasis
D) Inadequate development of the infant's respiratory center

Question 82: **If the infant turns red and cries, at what level of readiness to nurse would they be?**
A.   Medium cue
B.   Most cue
C.   Quick cue
D.   Late cue

Question 83: **What is the most important factor for the mother to maintain lactation?**
A.   Nipple inversion
B.   Mensural changes
C.   Nutrition
D.   Effective removal of milk from the breast

Question 84: **If the mother is obese, which of the following is NOT a risk factor?**
A. Food addiction/ Milk Addiction
B. Preterm delivery.
C. Fetal macrosomia.
D. None of the above.

Question 85: **Choose the correct answer. MRA is abbreviated as?**
A. Maternal Risk Assessment.
B. Maternal Role Attainment.
C. Management and Real Association.
D. Measurement Rapid Assessment.

Question 86: **What would be the normal dosage of oxytocin if administered IV to treat postpartum bleeding?**
A. 125 to 200 milliunits/minute
B. 700 to 950 milliunits/minute
C. 20 to 40 milliunits/minute
D. 5000 to 6500 milliunits/minute

.

Question 87: Jessica a 29-year-old female is in her 38th week of pregnancy. She is experiencing the second stage of labor. She is at low risk. To assess the overall well-being of the fetus how often do you auscultate for the fetal heart rate?

A. Every 5 minutes
B. Every 15 minutes
C. Every 45 minutes
D. Every 10 minutes

Question 88: A pregnant lady at 20 weeks of gestation came with complaints of fever (101 degrees Fahrenheit) and the following findings :

- Maternal tachycardia that is 110 beats per minute
- Fetal tachycardia 170 beats
- On examination, there was utero fundal tenderness

These findings suggest that this could be a case of chorioamnionitis. What are the risk factors leading to this condition?

A. Urinary tract infection
B. Syphilis
C. Preterm rupture of membrane
D. All of the above

Question 89: In a bedridden patient, deep vein thrombosis (DVT) in the lower limbs and abdomen are examined for all of the following EXCEPT?

A) Raised heart rate
B) Circulatory findings
C) Painful, edematous regions in the body
D) Raised temperature

Question 90: What is the congenital anomaly which has a more male preponderance (M: F=2:1) and is more common on the ankles and foot ?

A) Varicose veins
B) Dermoid cyst
C) Club foot
D) Fracture of the first metatarsal joint

Question 91: Choose the correct answer. Uterine involution does not involve which of the following?

A. Weight loss of at least 30 pounds.
B. Healing of the placental site through exfoliation without scarring.
C. Muscle fibers of uterus contraction leading to reduced stretch.

D. Regeneration of the epithelium of the uterus from the lower layer of decidua.

Question 92:   Mother of a newborn has a doubt of when the anterior fontanelle of her infant will close?
A.   9-18 months of age.
B.   0-6 months of age.
C.   6-12 months of age.
D.   1-2 months of age.

Question 93:   Which of the following is considered to have an effect on the developing fetus?
A. Teratogens
B. NSAID's.
C. Antibiotics.
D. Anti-diuretics.

Question 94:   How would the consistency of the infant's cranial sutures be felt?
A) Soggy
B) Nodular
C) Soft
D) Firm and flat

Question 95:   Casey a pregnant mother recently delivered and has experienced a 'postpartum chill'. What interventions will be adequate?
A) Administer beta blockers
B) Do a pre vaginal examination
C) Warm blankets
D) Get a chest X-ray done

Question 96:   Which of the following is the correct term that would describe the number of weeks after fertilization?
A. Baby age.
B. Fertilization age.
C. Ultrasound age.
D. Infant age

Question 97:   How long does it typically take for the posterior fontanelle of an infant to close?
A.   2 months or even before.

B.   5 months
C.   7 months
D.   9 months

Question 98:   In the hospital, a newborn is with a blood group B negative. The baby is at risk of hemolytic jaundice. Which of the following blood group will the mother be, that could be incompatible?
A. A+
B. A-
C. B+
D. O-

Question 99:   Which is NOT the effect of alcohol on the developing or unborn baby?
A. Decreases the RBC of the baby.
B. Alcohol crosses the placenta and reaches the infant.
C. Decreases the oxygen reaching the unborn baby.
D. Metabolizing alcohol takes more time in the infant

Question 100:   All of the following are true with regards to fetal tachysystole EXCEPT?
A.   Its prime focus is the frequency of contraction
B.   It is the condition wherein the contractions are closely separated out and seen at the time   of participation
C.   Both A and B
D.   It is related to a decrease in uterine contractions

Question 101:   A newborn in the maternity ward is seen to have 60 breaths per minute. Which of the following will describe the term?
A.   Tachypnea.
B.   Hypoventilation
C.   Tachycardia
D.   Bradypnea

Question 102:   Choose the correct answer. In case of uterus infection, which of the following is considered?
A. Chorioamnionitis
B. Microcarditis.
C. Metritis.

D. Endometritis.

Question 103: Select the right answer and most appropriate explanation for the following statement. "A normally fertilized ovum has 46 chromosomes.".
A)   The statement is incorrect as the fertilized ovum has 47 chromosomes
B)   The statement is correct, the fertilized ovum has 46 chromosome
C)   The statement is incorrect, the fertilized ovum has 48 chromosomes
D)   None of the above

Question 104: A patient is having a condition called placenta accrete. Which of the following is NOT true about the condition?
A. Identified during the blood work of 1st trimester.
B. Identified during a regular ultrasound examination.
C. Often no symptoms or signs.
D. Vaginal bleeding during the 3rd trimester.

Question 105: In case of prolapsed cord, which of the following symptoms might occur?
A. Fetal monitor shows fetal distress.
B. Mother may feel the cord.
C. Both A and B
D. Fever

Question 106: As a newborn transfer from intrauterine to extrauterine, which system undergoes multiple changes?
A.   Cardiorespiratory
B.   Adrenal
C.   Cholestatic
D.   Caudal

Question 107: Among the following which is the most common complication associated with hepatic rupture?
A.   Hypoglycemia
B.   Hypovolemic shock
C.   Hepatic hematoma
D.   None of the above

Question 108: Choose the correct answer for the abbreviation of NST.
A. Non-Stress Test.
B. Nose Stress Therapy

C. Neonatal System Therapy

D. New Stress Test.

Question 109: **A patient at 36 weeks gestation experiences pain in the right upper quadrant, has headache and pain in epigastric region. Lab results show elevated ALP and AST. Her systolic blood pressure and spasmodic pressure are elevated beyond normal. What would be your diagnosis based on the above findings?**

A.   Preeclampsia

B.   Abruptio placenta

C.   Rh incompatibility

D.   None of the above

Question 110: **When is an ECMO (extracorporeal membrane oxygenation) used?**

A. Persistent pulmonary hypertension.

B. Preterm labor

C. Placenta accreta

D. Asthma

Question 111: **Tina had carried three pregnancies to full term. Which term would be considered to describe this?**

A) Still birth

B) Para

C) Abortion

D) Death

Question 112: **Early deceleration occurring due to uterine contraction is caused by _____?**

A) Stimulation of the vagus nerve (vagal response)

B) The blood vessels are compressed

C) Release of epinephrine

D) Both a and c

Question 113: **Which is NOT an indication of postpartum C – section infection?**

A) Formation of a hematoma

B) Absence of pyrexia

C) Odor

D) Erythema

Question 114: Genelia is considered to be post-term and is suggested to undergo the C-section. When is pregnancy considered to be post-term?
A. More than 40 weeks of gestation
B. More than 42 weeks of gestation
C. More than 34 weeks of gestation
D. More than 38 weeks of gestation

Question 115: Lily, a 30-year-old female is 31 weeks pregnant. She is showing symptoms of uncontrolled asthma that may cause several fetal problems except for

_____.
A. Toxemia (Preeclampsia)
B. Retarded mental growth
C. Still birth
D. Pre term birth

Question 116: Rosie is a postpartum woman. Her uterus has not yet involuted. Which of the following factors play a role in it?
A) Size and weight of the placenta
B) Breastfeeding
C) Rapid ambulation
D) Birth without complications

Question 117: A woman who delivered the infant within 3 hours of the onset of contraction has what type of delivery?
A. Precipitous
B. Protracted
C. Retracted
D. Sudden

Question 118: The function of brown adipose tissue in a newborn is?
A) Hemopoiesis
B) Thermoregulation
C) Production of clotting factors
D) Source of red cell destruction

Question 119: Which of the following is not a characteristic of Fragile X syndrome?
A) Cardiac anomalies

B) Elongated face

C) Small ears

D) Diminished muscle tone

Question 120: A patient has blood pressure above 140/90 mm of hg in her readings prior to pregnancy. She is diagnosed to have?

A) Primary hypertension

B) Secondary hypertension

C) Chronic hypertension

D) White coat hypertension

Question 121: Which of the following could be a cause for the prolonged pregnancy?

A. Diabetes

B. Malnutrition

C. Low estrogen level during a normal pregnancy.

D. Smoking

Question 122: Which among the following is not indicated for assessing the fetal well-being

A.   Fetal heart monitoring

B.   Biophysical profile

C.   Fetal Doppler

D.   Kick counts of Fetus

Question 123: When can the internal fetal monitoring be performed?

A. After the amniotic sac rupture.

B. After the cervix has dilated to 2 cm.

C. After the amniotic sac has ruptured and the cervix has dilated to at least 4 cm.

D. None of the above.

Question 124: Which of the following must be considered while examining the post-partum mother's breast?

A. Color.

B. Size.

C. Weight.

D. Skin breakouts.

Question 125: Salpingitis/oophoritis refers to?

A) Inflammation of the vulva

B) Inflammation of mackenrodt's ligament

C) Inflammation of the cervix and ovaries

D) Inflammation of Fallopian tubes/ovaries

Question 126: **What is the term given to the thick substance which is waxy in nature and is present between fetal skin and amniotic sac?**

A) Amniotic fluid

B) Yolk sac

C) Vernix

D) Lanugo

Question 127: **A patient delivered a baby a few hours ago. During the post-partum period, the uterus fails to contract. What is this serious condition called?**

A. Uterine infection.

B. Uterine atony.

C. Post-partum infection.

D. Post-partum depression.

Question 128: **After delivery, what should the state of the uterus be?**

A.   Firm.

B.   Intense.

C.   Easy-going

D.   Inexhaustible.

Question 129: **What is the full form of PPH?**

A) Primitive Pontine Hemorrhage

B) Primary Pancreatic Hemorrhage

C) Primary Pontine Hemorrhage

D) Post Partum Hemorrhage

Question 130: **A pregnant patient has a history of drug abuse during her pregnancy. Her child is likely to have which among the following conditions?**

A) Neonatal abstinence syndrome

B) Neonatal-associated syndrome

C) Narcotic-associated syndrome

D) Narcotic abstinence syndrome

Question 131: **Fetal tachycardia is mostly seen due to?**

A) Maternal fever

B) Maternal thyrotoxicosis

C) Maternal anemia

D) Gestational diabetes

Question 132: A mother who is in the 20th week of gestation is found to be hypertensive. It might cause all except which of the following?
A.   Improve the oxygen supply to the fetus
B.   Abruptio placenta
C.   Hepatic rupture
D.   Miscarriage

Question 133: A mother is breastfeeding a newborn infant. Which of the following is the reflex that stimulates the cells of the breast muscle to eject the milk out?
A. Let-down reflex.
B. Star-up reflex.
C. Free Flow reflex.
D. Auto Flow Reflex

Question 134: A pregnant lady, 9 weeks into gestation is found to have a deformed fetus on an ultrasound scan. It is likely to cause all but which of the following in the neonate?
A.   Microcephaly
B.   Dislocation of the hip
C.   Clubbing of feet
D.   Preterm birth

Question 135: Ella 38 weeks pregnant is in labor. Which of the following would be considered a risk factor for the fetus during parturition
A.   Uncontrolled asthma
B.   Fetal head compression
C.   Hypoglycemia
D.   Seizures

Question 136: Ellie 26-year-old woman, 18 weeks of gestation presents with the following complaints:
- severe nausea
- vomiting
- dehydration
- anxiety
- morning sickness. This is most likely a case of _____ ?
A.   Food poisoning

B.   Hyperemesis gravidarum
C.   Morning sickness
D.   Bacteremia

Question 137:   Packed red blood cells (pRBCs) contain how much volume of blood?
A) 180ml
B) 200ml
C) 250ml
D) 500ml

Question 138:   Which of the following organisms cause UTI (urinary tract infection)?
A. Pneumonia
B. Virus.
C. Fungi
D. Bacteria.

Question 139:   The umbilical cord acts as conducting passage between the fetus and placenta and it is contained within Wharton's jelly. Which among the following is true about the umbilical cord?
A.   Wharton's Jelly supplies blood to Placenta
B.   Wharton's Jelly envelops the umbilical cord, provides cushioning effect, and protects the umbilical cord
C.   Umbilical cord has one vein and one artery
D.   Umbilical cord is not a part of the fetus initially

Question 140:   Which of the following would be considered a perforation of the uterus caused by the placenta?
A.   Placenta abruption
B.   Placenta increta
C.   Placenta previa
D.   Placenta percreta

Question 141:   A 28-year-old woman, at 34 weeks of gestation presents with severe abdominal pain and tachycardia. It was seen that there was fetal tachycardia. This is a most likely case of
A.   Latrogenic perforation.
B.   Polyhydramnios
C.   Uterine rupture
D.   Hypovolemia.

Question 142: A fetus in the mother's womb can be affected by a condition called Listeriosis. What is the possible way of harm that can occur to the fetus?
A. Fetal vision problems
B. Cerebellar Palsy.
C. Psychological disabilities.
D. Miscarriage and early delivery.

Question 143: A patient is a 39-year-old female. She is pregnant and since she is in her late stage of pregnancy, which of the options is not a complication of oligohydramnios?
A. Death of the fetus.
B. Weight of the fetus.
C. Preterm Delivery
D. Growth restriction of Fetus

Question 144: Which of the following test will be considered to determine if the postpartum patient has developed DVT (deep vein thrombosis)?
A. CT Scan of the lower extremities.
B. Doppler ultrasound of the lower extremities.
C. FMRI of lower extremities.
D. All of the above.

Question 145: Mariyah who is into her 39th week of pregnancy is in the active phase of labor. What would be the pattern of contractions that she will be experiencing?
A.   10 or fewer contractions in 10 minutes that lasts for about 90 seconds
B.   10 or fewer contractions in 10 minutes that lasts for about 60 seconds
C.   5 or fewer contractions in 10 minutes that lasts for about 60 seconds
D.   15 or fewer contractions in 10 minutes that lasts for about 60 seconds

Question 146: Nurse notices the position of a newborn Joe Brown, where his head turns to one side with his corresponding arm stretched out and opposite arm to bend at the elbow. Choose the correct term for this position.
A.   Palmar grasp.
B.   Tonic neck reflex.
C.   Plantar grasp.
D.   Suck reflex.

Question 147: The newborn attachment behavior period does not include which of the following?
A) Self-esteem of the mother
B) Financial status of the mother
C) Mother's trust
D) Mother's reaction to the present pregnancy

Question 148: The term given to define sporadic uterine contractions is called _____?
A) Peristalsis
B) Bruit
C) Thrill
D) Afterpains

Question 149: A patient in the hospital is suffering from bacterial vaginitis. Which of the following statement is not true considering bacterial vaginitis?
A. Sexually transmitted disease.
B. In the US, more than 1 million pregnant ladies suffer from BV every year.
C. The disease can be caused by the mother using the douching items.
D. This disease may increase the risk of premature birth.

Question 150: A patient is diagnosed with placenta previa without bleeding. How can it be treated after the 20th week of pregnancy?
A. Immediate medical attention.
B. Emergency normal delivery.
C. Emergency C-section.
D. Increase bed rest and low physical activity.

Question 151: Amelia a 28-year-old woman is one week into her postpartum, she had delivered the infant by C-section. Her bowel sounds will more likely be heard on which day?
A.   Day 3
B.   Day 4
C.   Day 5
D.   Day 6

Question 152: A Rh-negative mother is pregnant with her second child who is Rh-positive. The fetal heart sounds are showing a smooth regular pattern that resembles a wave. What do you conclude from the above-stated information?
A) The recorded wave pattern is sinusoidal and is indicative of Rh incompatibility

B) The wave pattern is sinusoidal and is indicated severe fetal anemia
C) Both a and b
D) The wave-particle is sinusoidal and is normal

Question 153: Which of the following food should not be avoided during pregnancy?
A. Hot dogs.
B. Luncheon meats.
C. Raw fruits.
D. Raw sprouts.

Question 154: Erica who is 34 weeks pregnant has gestational diabetes mellitus. The complication that cannot be anticipated is:
A. Still birth
B. Miscarriage
C. Hypoglycemia
D. Abruptio placenta

Question 155: What do you understand by zero station in association with labor?
A) The baby's head is known to be engaged or aligned with the ischial spine
B) The baby has descended beyond ischial spines
C) The baby's head is not engaged
D) None of the above

Question 156: Ultrasound scanning is performed _____ in pregnant women?
A. Transabdominal
B. Transurethral
C. Transvaginal
D. Both a and c

Question 157: All of the following are true about cervical insufficiency except?
A. Cervix is closed and is firm
B. Also called cervical Incompetence
C. It appears between 14 to 20 weeks of pregnancy
D. Fatal to the baby

Question 158: Which is the right term in the options given below for extra noise that is created when the mother and baby are moving together?
A. Artifact.

B. Fundus.

C. Audio.

D. Presentation.

Question 159: Which of the following number of chromosomes are considered abnormal leading to genetic defects?

A. Aneuploidy.

B. Periodicity

C. Transabdominal.

D. Polyploidy

Question 160: Children and newborns with cleft palates are at a higher risk of developing the following conditions:

A. Sight oedipus.

B. Anaphylaxis

C. Infections of the middle ear

D. Autism

Question 161: Which of the following is not at risk for placenta previa?

A. Surgical scarring to the uterus.

B. Large placenta, especially in multiple births.

C. No earlier pregnancy or uterine surgeries.

D. 35 years or older during pregnancy.

Question 162: A baby that is born after 40 weeks of gestation weighs 4 pounds and while comparing with average weight is of low birth weight. Among the following, all are contributory factors EXCEPT :

A. Smoking

B. Premature labor

C. Gonorrhea

D. Malnourished mother

Question 163: Which of the following is not a risk during the postpartum period?

A. Kidney failure.

B. Infection.

C. Hemorrhage.

D. Shock.

Question 164: HIPAA regulations require medical professionals to adhere to the regulations. This is termed as _____ :

a) Fidelity.
b) Validity.
c) Contract.
d) Slander.

Question 165: An ultrasound test is usually conducted with other tests to diagnose polyhydramnios. Which of the following test is used to diagnose polyhydramnios?

A. Urinalysis.
B. Glucose test.
C. CT Scan
D. Microscopy

Question 166: In which of the following, can a newborn infant lose body heat through convection?

A. Cold feet
B. During Bath
C. Cold Touch
D. Cool air vents.

Question 167: Are there any other terms for stretch marks that you would consider?

A.   Hemorrhage
B.   Striae
C.   Ovulation
D.   Evolution

Question 168: What is the most common variety of cord prolapse?

A) Funic
B) Overt
C) Occult
D) Paraumblical

Question 169: What is the abbreviation for VBAC?

A. Vaginal Blockage After Cesarean.
B. Vaginal Birth After Culture

C. Vaginal Birth After Cesarean.

D. Vaginal Bleeding After Cesarean.

Question 170:   The ectoderm, mesoderm, and endoderm are made by a biological process called _____ ?

A. Gastrulation.

B. Protostome

C. Blastocoel

D. Biploblastic

Question 171:   A neonate delivered at home 28 hours earlier shows the following symptoms: red and swollen eyes, and thick purulent discharge from the eyes. On staining the samples obtained from the discharge confirm the presence of Neisseria gonorrhea. Which among the following will you administer?

A.   Erythromycin

B.   Rifampicin

C.   Atenolol

D.   Streptomycin

Question 172:   A woman who is 20 weeks into gestation has hemoglobin values of nine grams per deciliter and laboratory tests also reveal a low serum iron and an increase in the total iron binding capacity suggestive of iron deficiency and anemia. There is an increased risk of?

A.   Preterm birth and low birth weight

B.   Still birth

C.   Retarded growth of fetus

D.   Fetal hepatic dysfunction

Question 173:   Doppler ultrasound is performed to assess the fetal heart rate and development of organs. It is indicated after how many months of pregnancy?

A.   1 month

B.   3 months

C.   4 months

D.   5 months

Question 174:   On performing fetal Doppler ultrasound the heart rate is found to be 180 beats per minute which is considered to be tachycardia, among the following what may lead to tachycardia?

A.   Exposure to beta-agonists

B.   Maternal hyperthyroidism
C.   Exposure to cocaine
D.   All of the above

Question 175: What is the normal range of the amniotic fluid?

A. 8 to 18 cms

B. 6 to 16 cms

C. 4 to 14 cms

D. None of the above.

Question 176:   National Council of States Boards of Nursing (NCSBN) is set up to carry out which functions?

A) Amendments to rules and regulations

B) Address loopholes in the law

C) To develop NCLEX RN and PN licensing exam

D) To approve clinical trials

Question 177:   As a nurse what role do you play in EFM?

A.   You need to inform the patient of the cost and make sure the payment is made.

B.   You need to explain to the patient the need for this treatment

C.   Required to record the results of EFM

D.   Both B and C

Question 178:   A woman who is 30 weeks pregnant shows the following symptoms: burning during maturation, and cloudy and smelly urine. Both of these are suggestive of urinary tract infection. There is an increased risk of which of the following?

A.   Preterm birth

B.   Stunted growth of the fetus

C.   Fetal hepatic dysfunction

D.   All of the above

Question 179:   State the time period for the mother's milk to "come in" after delivery of the baby?

A. 4-8 days.

B. 10-14 days.

C. 3-4 days.

D. Immediately.

Question 180:   A healthy neonate's anterior fontanelle is?
A) Diamond and open shaped
B) Oval and depressed
C) Triangular and elevated
D) Diamond and elevated

Question 181:   From the following, which is the important part that is included in the maternal pelvis?
A. Pelvic outlet.
B. Pelvic inlet
C. Pelvic block
D. Pelvic boundary

Question 182:   During labor, what is the percentage of fetal oxygen saturation that drops down?
A. 10.
B. 15.
C. 20.
D. 25.

Question 183:   Involution is known to be slowed by all factors, EXCEPT:
A. Infusion of anesthesia
B. Infection
C. Full bladder
D. Empty urinary bladder.

Question 184:   A baby's mother is suffering with a condition of lupus. This condition may lead to premature birth along with which of the following?
A) Neonatal Anemia
B. Neonatal Asthma
C. Neonatal thalassemia
D. Neonatal lupus.

Question 185:   If the normal uterine resting tone is 20 mm hg what is the conclusion?
A) It is the normal resting tone
B) It is borderline high and requires evaluation
C) It is normal resting tone during labor
D) Both a and b

Question 186:   Choose the correct answer. An infant has how many levels of cues when the infant is ready to nurse?

A. 1

B. 3

C. 2

D. None.

Question 187:   Which of the following degrees of episiotomies does not include?

A. Fifth degree.

B. Sixth degree.

C. Third degree.

D. First degree.

Question 188:   What is Homan's sign?

A.   Calf pain when the foot is dorsiflexed

B.   Back pain.

C.   Exercising causes pain in the upper back.

D.   Ankle pain in the right foot.

Question 189:   While evaluating the overall health of the fetus using the biophysical variables you will evaluate for all but which of the following?

A.   Tone of fetus

B.   Fetal movements

C.   Composition of amniotic fluid

D.   Organomegaly

Question 190:   On performing fetal Doppler ultrasound it is seen that there is changing baseline heart rate of the fetus and a recurrent decrease in the fetal heart rate following the sinusoidal path. Which category is this assigned to?

A.   Category 3

B.   Category 4

C.   Category 2

D.   Category 1

Question 191:   Which of the following is not considered to be the combination of Lochia?

A. Bone marrow.

B. Epithelial cells.

C. Fragments of decidua.

D. Mucus.

Question 192:   The normal fetal heart rate is 110-160 beats per minute. A Doppler ultrasound reveals a fetal heart rate above 160 beats per minute. This condition is termed as?

A.   Tachycardia
B.   Tachypnea
C.   Ventricular arrythmia
D.   Bradycardia

Question 193:   During the postpartum period, the mothers are asked to continue the prenatal vitamins. What is the reason?

A. Circulates airflow.
B. Maternal blood rebuilding
C. Stay Healthy
D. None of the above.

Question 194:   Nubain is a supplement for anesthesia. However, it was discontinued later. What was the reason for this?

A.   It may cause maternal dysphoria
B.   The drug was too expensive
C.   The supply could not meet the demands
D.   Limited nausea

Question 195:   In a patient who has developed abruptio placentae, which intervention would be less likely to be included?

a) Pitocin should be started at a higher dose for the patient
b) Provide oxygen to the patient
c) C-section the baby
d) Fluids should be administered via IV

Question 196:   Among the following which are true regarding abruptio placenta?

A.   It is the separation of the placenta from the womb
B.   There is intense abdominal pain, tender uterus, backache
C.   There is formation of Hematoma
D.   All of the above

Question 197: For the identification of PKU babies, the American Academy of Pediatrics recommends rescreening at which age after the first screening is performed within the first 24 hours of life. (PKU- inborn metabolism error).

A. 2-3 weeks.
B. 1-2 months.
C. 1-2 weeks.
D. 6 months.

Question 198: A patient complains of swollen and painful joints. He also complains of shortness of breath. On laboratory examination, it was confirmed to be Sickle Cell disease. What is true about Sickle Cell disease among the following?

A. The shape of red blood cells is affected
B. It is an inherited condition
C. Can be determined by prenatal screening of genetic trait
D. All of the above

Question 199: A woman who is 28 weeks into a pregnancy is asked to assess for fetal kicks. Which among the following is true about fetal kick/fetal kick evaluation?

A. Glucose is utilized by the fetus
B. It is due to the triggering of the autonomic nervous system
C. Indicator of the fetal distress
D. Development of normal muscle tone

Question 200: Protracted or prolonged labor is a condition where contractions are too weak. It has which of the following characteristics:

A. Slow dilation of the cervix
B. Early developing labor
C. Normal labor
D. Rapid dilation of the cervix

Question 201: What are the complications of post-term pregnancy?

A. Meconium aspiration
B. Cord complications
C. Peripheral nerve injury
D. All of the above

Question 202: What could be the most probable complication post-delivery?

A) Tenderness
B) Contusions
C) Hemorrhage

D) Dehydration

Question 203: Cell saver devices perform which of the following functions?
A.   Filters patients' blood
B.   Refiltration
C.   Infuses back
D.   All of the above

Question 204: From the below-given options, the maternal hypotension can lead to which of the following?
A. Early decelerations.
B. Rupture of membranes.
C. Dysrhythmias.
D. Uteroplacental insufficiency.

Question 205: Which of the following urinary signs should not be reported?
A. Clear color of the urine.
B. Urinary urgency.
C. Burning sensation while urination.
D. Retention of the urine.

Question 206: Bowel are assessed post-delivery for all the following EXCEPT?
A) Stool form
B) Restoration of bowel function
C) Color and consistency
D) Bowel sounds

Question 207: Physical signs of substance abuse is _____?
A. Low nutritional status
B. Hypoglycemia
C. High-risk sexual behavior.
D. Suicidal gestures.

Question 208: When the left side of the heart does not form correctly in the womb, it is called which of the following congenital birth defects?
A.   Hypoplastic left heart syndrome
B.   Coronary heart disease
C.   Tetralogy of fallot
D.   I-transposition of the great valves

Question 209: When the uterus is palpated after delivery, the highest point would be considered _____?

A. Tilt head
B. Fundus
C. Hotspurs
D. Branch

Question 210: Which of the following events will not be reportable by the patient to the state?

A. Patient protection events
B. Errors in Surgical Site
C. Wrong billing code.
D. Environmental Mishaps

Question 211: In which of the following women, afterpains are more common?

A) Women with BMI > 30
B) Woman who delivered only once
C) Multiparous women
D) Nulliparous

Question 212: What separates mitochondrial ATP synthesis from oxidative metabolism to create heat?

A. Bile
B. Brown adipose tissue
C. food products
D. Lungs

Question 213: Among the following, all are true about intrauterine resuscitation except.

A. It is performed to increase oxygen supply to the fetus
B.   The mother must be placed in a lateral recumbent position administering oxygen at 8 to 104 mm via a mask
C. It is used to treat hypoxia and reverse acidosis.
D. It measures the fetal metabolic rate

Question 214: Ollie was diagnosed with a parvovirus B19 infection (fifth disease) which is a common childhood disease. She is now pregnant, how does it affect her baby?

A) It is a self-limiting disease without any manifestations
B) It damages the fetal lymphatic system
C) It affects the fetal RBCs
D) Its effects on the fetus are still unknown

Question 215:   A fetus that has been exposed to promethazine in the womb shows bradycardia. Which among the following options also causes bradycardia?
A.   Metabolic acidosis
B.   While the fetus is asleep
C.   Drugs like opiates
D.   All of the above

Question 216:   If the PaO2 in the arterial blood gas results for a nonpregnant woman should be 90 to 100. What is the PaO2 that would be considered normal in a pregnant woman?
A) 110 to 114
B) 104 to 108
C) 120 to 139
D) 106 to 110

Question 217:   Nipple stimulation as a way to perform the contraction stress test is unreliable. What is the explanation for this?
A.   Nipple stimulation causes the release of oxytocin, and it cannot be controlled since it is released naturally.
B.   Nipple stimulation is a reliable way to induce labor
C.   Oxytocin released during nipple stimulation is not enough
D.   Both a and c

Question 218:   Which of the following is an acronym for EDD?
A.   Estimated Distribution of Disease
B.   Estimated Delivery Diagnosis
C.   Estimated Date of Delivery
D.   Evolution of Distribution of Delivery

Question 219:   A neonate Alice, has lost half a pound two days after delivery. Which of the following is true with respect to this?
A. It is normal
B. Vitamin D deficiency.
C. May cause fever
D. Acrocyonosis.

Question 220:   Elsa, a 37-year-old woman is a Prima gravida, complains of spontaneous abdominal pain. She is found to be hypertensive and on surgical intervention uterine rupture was found to be the cause. What are the ways in which it can be treated?

A.   Laparotomy
B.   C section
C.   Hysterectomy
D.   All of the above

Question 221:   Which of the following condition causes late hemorrhaging in the post-partum patient?
A. Uterine atony.
B. Bronchitis.
C. Viral Infection.
D. Blood Pressure

Question 222:   There is a transient increase in the fetal heart rate during a vaginal examination . Is this a cause of concern? What is it called?
A.   It is normal and it is called acceleration
B.   It is normal and it is called deceleration
C.   it is not normal for fetal heart rate to rise during the examination
D.   Fetal heart rate is always

Question 223:   A woman, 39 weeks into gestation has vaginal candidiasis. She is in labor and there is a spontaneous rupture of the membranes. The fetus will likely have which of the following
A.   Thrush (Oral candidiasis)
B.   Conjunctivitis
C.   Urethritis
D.   Fluid loss

Question 224:   A woman is 12 weeks into her pregnancy notices bleeding and experiences miscarriage. On further investigation, the pregnancy is found to be ectopic. What percentage of these occur in the fallopian tube?
A.   50%
B.   80%
C.   75%
D.   95%

Question 225:   What is the device used to monitor fetal heart sounds?
A) Doppler ultrasound device
B) ECG
C) Renault stethoscope
D) Sphygmomanometer

Question 226: Daisy comes to the doctor for her regular scan. Which of the following score is used to rate the gestational age of a fetus?

A.   Ballard
B.   Mallard
C.   Wingspan
D.   All of the above

Question 227: A hospital nursery should maintain a humidity level of _____.

A.   55% to 85%
B.   45% to 75%
C.   30% to 60%
D.   5% to 15%

Question 228: Choose the correct option. Symptoms like red, swollen, inflamed fetal membranes belong to which of the bacterial infection?

A.   Chlamydia
B.   Thrush
C.   Chorioamnionitis (intra-amniotic infection).
D.   Group A Streptococcus(GBS).

Question 229: Bronchopulmonary dysplasia (BPD) typically occurs in which of the given options?

A. Cesarean section born infants
B. Infants who require a ventilator to be used
C. If the infant bloodstream has high concentrations of oxygen
D. If the baby has umbilical cord problems at the time of delivery.

Question 230: What are the uses of EFM?

A.   It is used to monitor the fetal heart rate
B.   It is used to monitor the fetal metabolic rate
C.   It is used to monitor uterine contractions
D.   Both a and c

Question 231: What is the significance of fetal hiccups?

A.   It is a form of breathing reflex
B.   It signifies that the fetus is active
C.   It has no significance
D.   It is indicative of fetal distress

Question 232: Anna, a 30-year-old woman in 34 weeks of gestation presents with the following complaints :

-irritation and itching in the vagina

-burning micturition

It is suggestive of candida albican infection. The drug of choice for treating this infection will be?

A.   Fluconazole
B.   Ampicillin
C.   Bacitracin
D.   Metronidazole

Question 233: Kate is still pregnant beyond her due date and has entered post-dated pregnancy. What will NOT be a complication she may incur?

A) Wrinkly patchy skin of the baby
B) Fever
C) Fetal agenesis
D) Cord compression

Question 234: A newly delivered mother loses between 10 and 12 pounds at first. This weight consists of which of the following?

A.   Bleeding
B.   Diarrhea
C.   Delivery of the placenta
D.   Irritation

Question 235: Mark the correct statement with respect to chicken pox in association with pregnancy.

A) Chickenpox cannot be detected in a pregnant female
B) Clinical features cannot be elicited
C) 1-2 women who contract chicken pox also contract pneumonia
D) Chicken pox is the most common infection contracted during pregnancy

Question 236: A newborn baby has a lump on the skull likely to be caused due to blood accumulating below the periosteum. Which of the following refers to this?

A.   Ramsay hunt
B.   Dystocia
C.   Molding
D.   Cephalohematoma.

Question 237: In a full-term infant, there appears a blotchy, red rash in the newborn's upper body. Which of the following is the appropriate word?

A. Acrocyonosis.
B. Cold sore
C. Erythema Toxicum
D. Erysipelas

Question 238: _____ is an irregular accumulation of cerebrospinal fluid in the brain, which is often associated with spina bifida

A.   Hydrocephalus
B.   Klinefelter
C.   Thalassemia
D.   Alkaptonuria

Question 239: In infants and young children, the open space in the skull is called _____.

A.   Fontanelles.
B.   Mesosfera
C.   Parietal.
D.   Spatial.

Question 240: A woman, 38 weeks of gestation is experiencing protracted labor. She is administered Oxytocin. What would be the function of Oxytocin in this case?

A.   Induction of labor
B.   Reduces fetal mortality
C.   Reduces maternal mortality
D.   To prevent the development of the hemolytic disease of the newborn

Question 241: An infant with CMV infection is found to have microcephaly. It is a condition where?

A.   Shoulders are longer than normal
B.   Arms are longer than normal
C.   Head is smaller than the normal circumference
D.   Lungs are larger

Question 242: When does Rh incompatibility happen?

A. Mother's first pregnancy.
B. Immune system of infant attacks the mother's system.

C. Mother is Rh negative and the infant is Rh positive.
D. Mother is Rh negative and infant is Rh negative.

Question 243: A pregnancy was terminated at 6 to 8 weeks of gestation which of the following organs would be seen in the fetus?

A)   Lung
B)   Brain
C)   Heart
D)   Both B and C

Question 244: Placenta is of utmost importance for the growth of the fetus. Among the following which functions are fulfilled by the placenta?
A.   Supplies nutrients to the fetus
B.   Prevents loss of fluids
C.   Prevents organomegaly
D.   Regulates fetal heart rate

Question 245: A neonate born 48 hours earlier shows convulsions, tremors, seizures and the history suggests that the baby has been exposed to opioids in womb. It is likely a case of neonatal abstinence syndrome. Among the following which is NOT used to assess the condition?
A.   By obtaining fetal's stool sample
B.   By obtaining fetal's urine sample
C.   By obtaining fetal blood sample
D.   Neonatal squamous cell test

Question 246: Lauren who is in the 39th week of her pregnancy is in labor. It is found during examination that there was fetal head compression, and fetus is showing fall in heart rate which is gradual and reaches back to the baseline, this is associated with uterine contraction. This is considered as _____.
A.   Intermittent deceleration
B.   Late deceleration
C.   Early deceleration
D.   Recurrent deceleration

Question 247: A woman who is suspected of molar pregnancy has hCG values 100000. The proposed plan of treatment will be?
A.   Termination of pregnancy
B.   Dilatation and curettage

C.   C section
D.   Treatment is not indicated

Question 248:   Placenta previa is a condition where the placenta covers the internal opening of the cervix. It can lead to complications like bleeding before or during parturition. Among the following what is the treatment for placenta previa?
A.   Blood transfusion
B.   Hospitalization of the patient
C.   C-section
D.   All of the above

Question 249:   An approximate initial weight loss for a new mother would be which of the following?
A.   5 to 8 pounds
B.   20 to 40 pounds
C.   10 to 12 pounds
D.   8 to 16 pounds

Question 250:   When the membranes rupture, how soon do contractions usually begin?
A. 5 to 10 hours.
B. 8 to 15 hours.
C. 12 to 48 hours.
D. 24 to 72 hours.

Question 251:   Choose the correct answer. Which of the following is covered by the childbirth classes?
A. Method of breathing.
B. Fees of classes.
C. Way of handling finances after the baby's birth.
D. None of the above.

Question 252:   Mona is regularly breastfeeding her baby. She wants to know when her periods will resume. The answer would be ?
A) 3weeks
B) 6 weeks
C) 12 weeks or more
D) 4 weeks

Question 253: A standard vital sign for a postpartum woman would be all but one of the following?

A. Breathing
B. Measurement of temperature
C. Rate of heartbeat
D. Weight

Question 254: Surfactant is detected in the amniotic fluid by 28 to 32 weeks, it is composed of which among the following?

A. Sphingomyelin
B. Calcitonin
C. Melatonin
D. Thyroxin

Question 255: Which among the following statements is correct

A. Fetal movements can be assessed after 28 weeks
B. Fetal movements can be assessed after 16 weeks
C. Fetal movements can be assessed between 14-18weeks
D. Fetal movements can be assessed after 19 weeks

Question 256: A patient is considered to have Placenta Accreta when the placenta is not delivered within how many minutes of delivery of the infant?

A. 5 minutes.
B. 30 minutes.
C. 35 minutes.
D. None of the above.

Question 257: Genital herpes can be passed on to an infant in certain ways. Which of the following is a cause of transmission for genital herpes?

A. Genetically.
B. Hereditary
C. Postpartum, by contact.
D. Chromosomal disorders.

Question 258: Geneva is diagnosed with mastitis. It indicates all the below EXCEPT:

A) Mastalgia
B) Edematous breasts

C) Empty breasts
D) Inflamed breasts

Question 259: Daisy has massive vaginal bleeding in her 3rd month of pregnancy. The cause was diagnosed to be placental abruption. Which type of abruptio placenta is it ?
A) Complete
B) Incomplete
C) Marginal
D) Circumvallate

Question 260: What is the full form of FRC ?
A) Full Resonance Capacity
B) Fatal Restoration Column
C) Functional Residual Capacity
D) Functional Resonance Capacity

Question 261: What is vibroacoustic stimulation?
A) It is placed over abdomen of mother and emits sounds at a level that is predetermined
B) It is used to measure fetal metabolic heart rate
C) Non invasive technique to obtain reassurance of fetal wellbeing
D) Both a and c

Question 262: Which of the following is not seen during the postpartum period?
A. Changes in the breast.
B. Lochia
C. Loss of hair.
D. Cervical involution.

Question 263: Nyla had delivered a healthy baby through a normal vaginal delivery with episiotomy. Which of the following includes good nursing interventions?
A) IV antibiotics
B) Sitz bath
C) Good pericare
D) B and C

Question 264: A symmetric fall in the heart rate of fetus following peak uterine contractions is called_____ ?
A) Early deceleration
B) Intermediate deceleration
C) Late deceleration

D) Acute deceleration

Question 265: A mother who has delivered shows the following symptoms: mood swings, depression, and mood disorder. The most probable diagnosis is _____ and it is linked to _____?
A.   Maternal depression, postpartum depression
B.   Hypoglycemia, lack of proper diet
C.   Sleep deprivation and Mood swings
D.   both a and b

Question 266: Which is NOT a non-pharmacological intervention to support a newborn with withdrawal symptoms?
A) Swaddling
B) Rocking
C) Bright room
D) Use of a pacifier

Question 267: Which of the following is the most abnormal presentation during pregnancy?
A. Occiput posterior presentation.
B. Face presentation.
C. All of the above.
D. None of the above.

Question 268: A baby is being monitored for fetal alcohol syndrome, which of the following must be assessed by the medical professional?
A. Puffy hands
B. Poor suck reflex.
C. Startle reflex
D. Hermaphrodite

Question 269: Select the correct option for NST. Which of the following is a disadvantage of NST (Non-Stress Test)?
A. Quicker.
B. Easy interpretation.
C. No side effects.
D. Often hard to obtain a required tracing.

Question 270: Choose the correct answer. Which of the following range gives us the correct value of maternal platelet count?

A. 150-400.

B. 60-120.

C. 150-400.

D. None of the above.

Question 271: What is the prevalence of polyhydramnios amongst pregnant women?

A.   4-6%

B.   1 -3%

C.   10-20%

D.   2-8%

Question 272: A patient is undergoing a C-section procedure in the Operation Theatre. For the Cesarean or C-section procedure, the head of the fetus is pushed back into the birth canal. What is this condition called?

A. Henry's maneuver.

B. Woods' scrape maneuver.

C. Zavanelli maneuver.

D. None of the above.

Question 273: In which of the following cervical cerclage is performed?

A. Incompetent cervix

B. Toxemia.

C. Septicemia

D. Preeclampsia

Question 274: During labor, how can broken bones occur?

A.   Birth assisting instruments

B.   C Section

C.   Tinea cruris

D. None of the above

Question 275: Cord blood gas analysis is performed when_____.

A) There is a risk of neonatal encephalopathy

B) The mother has a thyroid disorder

C) Both a and b

D) The fetus is overweight

Question 276: Choose the correct answer. Which of the following complication is considered most common in Placenta Previa?

A. Neurological problems.
B. Preterm birth.
C. Hyperglycemia.
D. Hypertension.

Question 277: A newborn born to a diabetic mother shows agenesis of the lumbar spine, sacrum, and coccyx .There is a hypoplasia of the lower extremities. What is the most probable diagnosis in this case?

A.   Phocomelia
B.   Caudal agenesis
C.   Radiation exposure
D.   None of the above

Question 278: A woman at 38 weeks of gestation is in labor. She delivers the infant in two hours after the onset of contractions. Her medical card states that this was precipitous labor. How long does labor last in precipitous labor?

A.   2-4 hours
B.   3-6 hours
C.   1-3 hours
D.   4-8 hours

Question 279: There are several types of tumors that can develop on the placenta, but the most common would be called _____.

A. Pressure ulcer
B. Choriocarcinoma
C. Metaplasia
D. Chorioangioma

Question 280: When does the acute fatty liver occur in a pregnant woman?

A. 1st trimester.
B. 2nd trimester.
C. 1st and 2nd trimester.
D. 3rd or immediately after delivery.

Question 281: Which of the following is not a mechanism of heat loss?

A) Condensation

B) Evaporation

C) Convection

D) Conduction

Question 282: Which of the following term must be considered when the uterus returns back to the non-pregnant state from the pregnant state?

A. Involution.

B. Convolution

C. Postpartum.

D. Pumping

Question 283: A pregnant woman given an epidural is showing the following symptoms: itchiness, nausea, vomiting and fainting. What is the most likely cause?

A) Hypoglycemia

B) Hyperglycemia

C) Hypotension due to epidural

D) None of the above

Question 284: Mrs.Maurice complained of sore nipples. What intervention would provide her with relief?

A) Ask her to withdraw breast feeding

B) Put the infant on solid foods

C) Check latching or baby's positioning

D) Do-not intervene

Question 285: Nina a pregnant woman, showed signs of early placental separation from the uterine wall much earlier than her due date. What is the condition ?

A) Placenta Previa

B) Abruptio placenta

C) Cervical incompetence

D) Vasa Previa

Question 286: A newborn is showing elevated liver enzymes and symptoms of hepatic rupture. He is considered to be in a surgical emergency. Which among the following is also a surgical emergency?

A.   Subscapular hematoma

B.   Hyperthermia

C. Hypoglycemia

D. Eroded skin

Question 287: **Which of the following is the outer layer of germ cells?**

A. Ectoderm.

B. Endoderm.

C. Cytoderm

D. Pectoderm

Question 288: **What is the biophysical score?**

A) Used to measure fetal health

B) Is a non-stress test

C) It is used to measure amniotic fluid

D) Both a and b

Question 289: **Nora is undergoing delivery and has been noted that her baby's presenting part is breech. How would you intervene in this case?**

A) Continue with normal vaginal delivery

B) Administer corticosteroids

C) Do Caesarean section

D) Give oxytocin

Question 290: 36-year-old female patient is showing the following symptoms:

- **Watery, creamy or greenish vaginal discharge**
- **pain or burning while urinating**
- **pain during penetrative vaginal intercourse**
- **heavier periods or spotting o**

What is the most probable diagnosis?

A. Syphilis

B. Gonorrhea

C. HIV

D. Yeast infection

Question 291: **In Gynecology, which of the following is not included in the ethical principles in nursing?**

A. Veracity

B. Justice.

C. Confidentiality

D.   Implementation.

Question 292:   Jessie was diagnosed with vulval hematoma. Which of the following are NOT used to treat it ?
A) Nifedipine
B) A surgical drain is made in the vulva
C) Initiate transfusion of blood
D) Ligation of bleeding vessels

Question 293:   Ultrasound scanning is performed _____ in pregnant women?
A.   Transabdominal
B.   Transurethral
C.   Transvaginal
D.   Both a and c

Question 294: It should be noted that all of the following symptoms are indicative of a vulval hematoma, except for:
A.   The vagina has been swelling steadily on one side.
B.   Shock associated with hemorrhage.
C.   Sitting down causes severe pain.
D.   Vaginal discharge that is severe

Question 295.   What would constitute the first hour postpartum?
A.   3rd stage
B.   1st stage
C.   4th stage
D.   5th stage

Question 296. How much percentage of the infant's body does a head form immediately after birth?
A. 25%.
B. 15%.
C. 30%.
D. 35%.

Question 297: Uterine involution means_____ ?
A. Decrease in muscle mass of the uterus
B. Gradual return of the uterus to its non pregnant size
C. Process by which the cervix and vagina regain their pre pregnant state
D. All of above

Question 298: Symptom of postpartum C – section infection is _____?
   A. Redness and swelling at the site
   B. Hypertension
   C. Diabetes mellitus
   D. Cataract

Question 299: Usually how long does it take for periods to resume after pregnancy?
 A)0-2 weeks
 B) 7-9 weeks
 C) 2-3weeks
 D) 3-4 weeks

Question 300: If you were to administer a medication for Neisseria gonorrhea to a newborn, which one would you choose?

 A.   Erythromycin
 B.   Rifampicin
 C.   Atenolol
 D.   Streptomycin

Answers with Explanation

Answers with Rationale For the Inpatient Obstetric Nurse

Question 1:

Answer: C. Americans with disabilities act (ADA)

Explanation: Federal civil rights legislation known as the Americans with Impairments Act (ADA) forbids discrimination against those with disabilities. The ADA covers all aspects of everyday life, including employment, education, transportation, and access to public places. The ADA also contains strict requirements for accommodating people with disabilities in all aspects of life. In the context of doctor's offices, the ADA requires that all medical offices make reasonable accommodations for people with disabilities. This means that doctor's offices must be designed in a way that is accessible to people with disabilities, and that staff must be trained to provide care in an accommodating way. There are a few specific accommodations that are often required in doctor's offices. One is the provision of accessible examination rooms. This means that the rooms must be large enough to accommodate a person in a wheelchair and that all of the equipment must be placed in an accessible manner. Another common accommodation is the use of assistive listening devices. These devices amplify sound so that people with hearing impairments can more easily hear what is being said.

Question 2:

Answer:

C. Aversion to certain foods

Explanation: An extrauterine pregnancy is referred to as an ectopic pregnancy. The most common location for an ectopic pregnancy is in the Fallopian tubes, but it can also occur in the ovary, cervix, or abdominal cavity. The most common symptom of an ectopic pregnancy is abdominal pain, typically on one side. Other signs and symptoms may include vaginal bleeding, shoulder pain (due to bleeding into the abdomen and irritating the diaphragm), and nausea or vomiting. Aversion to certain foods is not a sign of ectopic pregnancy.

Question 3:

Answer: D. All of the above

Preeclampsia is a condition that pregnant women can experience High blood pressure and protein in the urine are its defining symptoms. Preeclampsia can occur anytime after the 20th week of pregnancy and usually goes away after the baby is delivered. However, in some cases, it can lead to serious complications, such as seizures, organ damage, and even death. Preeclampsia comes in two forms: early-onset and late-onset. Early-onset preeclampsia occurs before the 34th week of pregnancy and is more likely to lead to serious complications. Late-onset preeclampsia occurs after the 34th week of pregnancy and is less likely to cause serious complications. Preeclampsia has a number of risk factors, including: * A family history of preeclampsia * Obesity * Diabetes * High blood pressure * Kidney disease . There is no one cause of preeclampsia.

Question 4:

Answer:

B. Endocervical os with placenta overlaying

Explanation: Placenta Previa is a condition that occurs during pregnancy. In this condition, the placenta grows in the lowest part of the womb or uterus that covers the entire or some portion at the opening of the cervix. The placenta feeds the developing baby that forms the attachment between the mother and the baby. The cervix forms the entrance of the birth canal.

Question 5:

Answer:
B.110 to 160 beats per minute

EXPLANATION: A normal fetal heart rate (FHR) usually ranges from 110 to 160 beats per minute (bpm). It is important to note that there is some variability in what is considered to be a normal FHR. For example, some sources may cite a normal range of 120-160 bpm. It is also important to keep in mind that the FHR can vary throughout the course of pregnancy, as well as during labor and delivery. The FHR can be determined by auscultation (listening with a stethoscope) or by electronic monitoring.

Question 6:

Answer:
A.   Pyrexia and symptoms suggestive of flu

EXPLANATION: Bacterial vaginosis (BV) is a mild infection of the vagina caused by bacteria. The symptoms of BV include a fishy-smelling discharge, burning during urination, and itching around the outside of the vagina. Pyrexia, or a fever, is not a symptom of BV. Instead, it is a symptom of another infection, such as the flu. Symptoms of the flu can include a fever, sore throat, coughing, and runny nose.

Question 7:
answer: option: C)preeclampsia
Explanation: The most probable diagnosis is preeclampsia. Preeclampsia is a pregnancy-related condition that can result in high blood pressure and protein in the urine. It can be a very serious condition and can lead to complications such as preterm labor, placental abruption, and low birth weight. If you one is diagnosed with preeclampsia, it is important to be closely monitored by a healthcare provider and to get regular checkups.

Question 8:

Answer:
D. Both B and C

Explanation: Magnesium sulfate is a medication that is used to treat a variety of conditions. One of the conditions that it is prescribed for is preeclampsia. High blood pressure and protein in the urine are symptoms of the condition known as preeclampsia, which can develop during pregnancy. Magnesium sulfate can help to prevent or treat preeclampsia. Another condition that magnesium sulfate is prescribed for is to reduce the risk of brain damage to the baby. Magnesium sulfate can help to prevent or treat eclampsia. Magnesium sulfate is also prescribed for preterm labor. Preterm labor is when labor starts earlier than 37 weeks into a pregnancy. Magnesium sulfate can help to stop or reduce the chances of preterm labor. Magnesium sulfate is also prescribed for gestational diabetes. One type of diabetes that can develop during pregnancy is gestational diabetes. Magnesium sulfate can help to control blood sugar levels in women with gestational diabetes.

Question 9:

answer) Option
A)Uterine Rupture
Explanation: A tear in the uterus's wall is known as a uterine rupture. Symptoms of a uterine rupture include abdominal pain, vaginal bleeding, and fetal bradycardia (slow heart rate). A uterine rupture is a serious complication of pregnancy and can lead to maternal and fetal death. Treatment of a uterine rupture includes emergency cesarean delivery and resuscitation of the mother and baby.

Question 10
answer) Option
B)0-8
Explanation) The International Society of Thrombosis and Hemostasis (ISTH) is a professional society dedicated to promoting research and education in the field of thrombosis and hemostasis. The ISTH offers a wide range of educational courses, from basic science to clinical practice, that are designed to meet the needs of both biomedical researchers and clinicians. The courses range from 0-8, with the higher number courses being more advanced. The ISTH also offers certification programs for those who wish to specialize in thrombosis and hemostasis. ISTH members are involved in all aspects of thrombosis and hemostasis, including venous and arterial thrombosis, thrombotic and hemorrhagic disorders in pregnancy, myocardial infarction, stroke and other cerebrovascular disease, thrombocytopenia and platelet function disorders, hemostasis and thrombosis in surgery, and laboratory methods for the diagnosis and management of thrombotic and bleeding disorders.

Question 11
Answer: D. All of the above
EXPLANATION: There are many reasons why a woman may opt for an elective C-section, but one common reason is prolonged labor. In this situation, the woman may be given Oxytocin to help speed up the delivery. Oxytocin is a hormone that is produced naturally in the body and it plays an important role in various bodily functions. In pregnant women, Oxytocin is released during labor to help the uterus contract and push the baby out. It is also in charge of breastfeeding's let-down reflex and also controlling hemorrhage. Some of the other functions of Oxytocin include: - Promoting bonding between people - Reducing anxiety -Regulating blood pressure -Stimulating the release of other hormones.

Question 12:

Answer: A. Malpractice

EXPLANATION. Medical malpractice is a legal term that describes a situation in which a healthcare provider negligently provides sub-standard care to a patient, resulting in harm. Malpractice can occur in any medical setting, including hospitals, clinics, nursing homes, and physicians' offices. There are four main elements to a medical malpractice claim: duty, breach, causation, and damages. The first element, duty, requires that the healthcare provider owed the patient a duty of care. The second element, breach, requires that the healthcare provider breached that duty of care. The third element, causation, requires that the breach of duty of care caused the patient's injury. The fourth and final element, damages, requires that the patient suffered some type of damage as a result of the injury.

Question 13:

Answer:

C. Crepitus.

Explanation: Crepitus is the grating or crackling sound that is produced when the ribs of a newborn are rubbed together. This is a result of the uneven cartilage growth in the newborn's ribs. The cartilage is not yet fully developed and is still growing at different rates. This causes the ribs to rub together and produces the characteristic crepitus sound. Crepitus is a normal finding in newborns and is nothing to be concerned about. It is not painful and will resolve on its own as the cartilage grows and matures.

Question 14:

Answer:

A. Surgery.

Explanation: Placental insufficiency is a condition that can occur when the placenta is not able to provide enough blood and nutrients to the developing fetus. This can happen for a variety of reasons, including preeclampsia, placental abruption, and intrauterine growth restriction. Surgery is not a direct cause of placental insufficiency.

Question 15:

answer: Option

D) 125 mg given in 100ml normal saline

Explanation: Sodium ferric gluconate is an iron supplement that is used to treat iron deficiency anemia. It is available in oral and injectable forms. The injectable form is given as an IV infusion. The recommended dose of sodium ferric gluconate for a pregnant woman is 125 mg given in 100 ml of normal saline. This dose is safe for use in pregnancy and has been shown to be effective in treating iron deficiency anemia.

Question 16:

Answer: D. Socio-economic status of the family

EXPLANATION: The maternal and fetal health evaluation process typically includes assessing the health of the mother and fetus from a physical standpoint. This usually includes things like checking for any physical abnormalities or birth defects, monitoring the mother's health during pregnancy, and testing the fetus for any genetic conditions that may be present. However, socio-economic status is not typically included as part of this evaluation process. There are a few potential reasons for this. For one, socio-economic status is not always a reliable predictor of health. There are many families of low socio-economic status who are perfectly healthy, and vice versa. Additionally, assessing socio-economic status can be quite subjective and difficult to quantify. As such, it can be a difficult factor to take into consideration when trying to assess someone's health.

Question 17

Answer :

B. Localized

Explanation

Scleroderma is a chronic, progressive autoimmune disease that affects the connective tissues and blood vessels of the body. It can be classified into two types: localized and systemic. Localized scleroderma is limited to the skin and not associated with any other organs. It is the most common type of scleroderma in children, and can often resolve on its own. Systemic scleroderma, on the other hand, can involve major organs such as the heart, lungs, and kidneys, and is often associated with Raynaud's phenomenon. Pregnancy can be complicated in women with scleroderma, particularly those with systemic disease. There is an increased risk for pre-eclampsia, gestational diabetes, and premature delivery. The is also a higher risk for perinatal mortality.

Question 18

Answer:

A. Deep vein thrombosis (DVT).

EXPLANATION: Dorsiflexion is the movement of the foot upwards towards the shin, while plantarflexion is the movement of the foot downwards away from the shin. The term 'dorsiflexion' is derived from the Latin word for 'backward', while 'plantarflexion' is derived from the Latin word for 'foot'. When a blood clot develops in a deep vein, commonly in the leg, DVT occurs. The clot can block the flow of blood and cause swelling and pain. Homans' sign is a DVT diagnosis method that involves pressing on the calf to see if pain occurs in the calf or foot. A positive Homans' sign indicates that there is likely a DVT present.

Question 19

Answer:

C. Umbilical cord compression for a long time

Explanation: When the umbilical cord is compressed for a long time, it can cause fetal bradycardia. This is because the umbilical cord is the baby's lifeline to the placenta and it delivers oxygenated blood to the baby. If the cord is compressed, it can't deliver as much oxygenated blood to the baby, which can cause the baby's heart rate to slow down. This can be dangerous for the baby and can lead to complications.

Question 20:

Answer:
D. Prior to placing the syringe tip into the infant's mouth, depress the bulb

Explanation: Cleaning the mucus from an infant's nose and mouth is an important part of keeping them healthy and free from infection. However, it is important to take care when doing this, as the syringe can easily accidentally enter the infant's airway. To prevent this, the nurse should first depress the bulb on the syringe. This will ensure that there is no air in the syringe, which could be forced into the infant's airway when the mucus is suctioned out. Once the bulb has been depressed, the nurse can then place the syringe tip into the infant's mouth. They should be careful to avoid the tongue and teeth and to only insert the tip a small way into the mouth. If the syringe is inserted too far, it could enter the infant's airway. Once the syringe is in place, the nurse can then release the bulb, which will allow the mucus to be suctioned out.

Question 21

Answer:
D. Shortness of breath.

Explanation: When most people think of a urinary tract infection (UTI), they think of the symptoms that are most commonly associated with the condition: a burning sensation when urinating, cloudy urine, and/or strong-smelling urine. However, there are other less common symptoms of a UTI that are important to be aware of. One of these less common symptoms is shortness of breath. While shortness of breath is not a symptom that is typically associated with a UTI, it can occasionally be a sign that the infection has spread to the lungs. This is more likely to occur in people who have a weakened immune system or other underlying health conditions.

Question 22:

Answer:
A. Bright yellow.

Explanation: When a baby is first born, its intestines are sterile and contain no bacteria. As they start to breastfeed, they begin to ingest bacteria from their mother's breast milk. This bacteria is vital for their development and helps them to break down and digest their food. The majority of a baby's stool is made up of this bacteria, which is why it is usually yellow. However, there may also be small amounts of meconium (the baby's first stool) and urine mixed in, which can change the color slightly.

Question 23:
Answer:
A. More than 8 cm maximum pool.

Explanation: Polyhydramnios is the condition where the amniotic fluid is excessive around the baby during pregnancy than the ideal amount. A large amount of amniotic fluid is normally spotted during a check-up in the later stages of pregnancy. The definition of polyhydramnios would include 2000 mL of amniotic fluid, more than 8 cm maximum pool, AFI more than 25 cm.

Question 24:

Answer :

B. 7-9 weeks

Explanation : When a woman delivers a baby, her body expels the placenta and the uterine lining, which stops her menstrual bleeding. For a non-lactating woman, it takes approximately seven to nine weeks for her period to resume. The first few postpartum periods may be irregular and heavier than usual. The hormone levels in a woman's body gradually return to normal after delivery, which can take several months.

Question 25:

Answer:

B. Placental abruption.

Explanation : The placenta is a crucial part of the pregnancy, providing oxygen and nutrients to the baby and helping to remove waste products. Placental abruption is a serious complication and can lead to the baby being born prematurely, or even stillborn.. It also produces hormones that help to maintain the pregnancy. A placental abruption is when the placenta starts to come away from the wall of the uterus before the baby is born. This can happen either partially or completely.   It can also cause heavy bleeding in the mother, which can be life-threatening. Placental abruption is more common in certain groups of women, including those who are smokers, are overweight, have high blood pressure, or have had a previous placental abruption. If you think you might be experiencing placental abruption, you should contact your doctor or midwife immediately.

Question 26:

answer) Option

A) Meconium plug syndrome

Explanation) Meconium plug syndrome is a condition where the meconium, a baby's first stool, is not passed. This can happen because the meconium is too thick, or there is a blockage in the intestine. This can be a problem because the meconium can cause an infection if it is not passed. Meconium plug syndrome is more common in premature babies, but it can happen in full-term babies as well. If your baby has meconium plug syndrome, the doctor will likely do a test called a barium enema to check for a blockage. If the blockage is resolved, your baby will likely be able to pass the meconium on its own. If the blockage is not resolved, your baby may need surgery to remove the blockage.

Question 27
Answer:

A.   The abdominal wall is weakened and muscle tone is diminished.

EXPLANATION: The abdominal wall is a layer of muscle and connective tissue that encircles the abdomen. It is supported by the pelvis, ribs, and spine. The abdominal muscles are responsible for most of the strength and stability of the abdominal wall. During pregnancy, the abdominal wall is weakened and muscle tone is diminished. This is due to the increased weight of the baby and the pressure of the expanding uterus on the muscles and connective tissue of the abdominal wall. The weakened abdominal muscles are unable to provide adequate support for the spine and pelvis, and the increased pressure on the abdominal organs can lead to back pain and other problems. To compensate for the weakened abdominal muscles, the pregnant woman must rely on her pelvic floor muscles and deep abdominal muscles to support her spine and pelvis. These muscles are also under increased strain during pregnancy and can become weak and stretched out. As the baby grows, the uterus puts pressure on the large veins in the abdomen, which can cause varicose veins.

Question 28:
Answer:

A.   Phenylketonuria

EXPLANATION: Phenylketonuria (PKU) is a metabolic disorder in which the body cannot break down the amino acid phenylalanine. This amino acid is found in all proteins, so people with PKU must follow a diet that is low in protein. Untreated, PKU can lead to seizures, mental retardation, and behavioral problems. The newborn screening process in the United States includes a test for PKU. This test is usually done when a baby is between 2 and 4 days old. A heel stick is used to collect a small sample of blood, which is then sent to a laboratory for testing. If the test shows that a baby has high levels of phenylalanine in his or her blood, the baby will be referred to a doctor who specializes in treating PKU. The diagnosis will be confirmed by additional tests. If PKU is diagnosed, the baby will need to be on a special diet. This diet is low in protein and high in a special amino acid called phenylalanine-hydroxylase.

Question 29:
Answer:

A.   Swaddling the infant tightly

EXPLANATION: The Neonatal Abstinence Syndrome (NAS) refers to a group of symptoms that may occur in newborns who are exposed to drugs while in the womb. These symptoms may include seizures and tremors, as well as irritability, poor feeding, and difficulty sleeping. NAS is typically treated with medication, but in some cases, swaddling the infant tightly may also be effective. Swaddling is a technique that involves wrapping the infant in a blanket or other piece of cloth so that the baby's arms and legs are immobilized. This can help to calm the baby and reduce the risk of self-injury. In cases of NAS, swaddling may be used in conjunction with medication to help control the symptoms. There is no one-size-fits-all approach to treating NAS, and the best course of treatment will vary depending on the individual situation. However, swaddling can be an effective way to provide comfort and stability for an infant with NAS.

Question 30:

answer) Option A) It is an excess of amniotic fluid seen mostly during the second trimester of pregnancy

Explanation:

Around the world, the average amount of amniotic fluid is approximately 800 ml. However, women can have anywhere from 500 mL to over 1,000 mL, and still, be within the "normal‿ range. Polyhydramnios, also called hydramnios, is a pregnancy complication that occurs when there is too much amniotic fluid surrounding the baby. In some cases, the cause is unknown. However, it can also be caused by certain birth defects, such as Down syndrome or congenital heart defects. It can also be caused by twins or triplets, a condition called twin-to-twin transfusion syndrome, infection, or Rh incompatibility (when the mother is Rh-negative and the baby is Rh-positive). Polyhydramnios can cause the baby to grow too large and become macrosomic (a baby that weighs more than 8 pounds 13 ounces at birth).

Question 31

Answer:
D. Velamentous cord insertion

EXPLANATION: When the blood vessels in the umbilical cord do not have Wharton's jelly to protect them, they are more susceptible to compression and damage. One of the most common complications associated with this is velamentous cord insertion, which occurs when the blood vessels cross the membranes before joining to form the cord. This can cause the cord to become kinked or twisted, and can ultimately lead to fetal demise. While this is a rare complication, it is one that can be avoided by ensuring that the blood vessels have adequate protection.

Question 32

Answer:
A.Asthma

EXPLANATION:" Depression during pregnancy can have a number of negative consequences for the developing infant. The most significant of these is probably the increased risk for preterm birth, which can lead to a host of problems including low birth weight, respiratory distress, and developmental delays. Additionally, infants born to mothers with depression are more likely to be born small for gestational age. Infants of mothers with depression are also at increased risk for a number of other problems. One of the most well-documented is deficits in social-emotional development. These babies are more likely to be irritable, cry more, and have difficulty self-regulating their emotions. They may also have difficulty forming attachments to their caregivers. Additionally, although the research is somewhat mixed, it appears that infants of depressed mothers are more likely to experience feeding problems and be at risk for developing obesity.

Question 33:

Answer:
B. Cervical incompetence.

Explanation: The cervix is the uterus' bottom, thin end. It opens into the vagina and during pregnancy, it is held closed by muscular and fibrous tissue. Cervical incompetence refers to a condition in which the cervix does not stay closed during pregnancy. This can lead to preterm labor and delivery, as well as pregnancy loss.   There are a number of factors that can contribute to cervical incompetence, including previous damage to the cervix, such as from previous childbirth or abortion; a weak or thin cervix; or hormones. The cause may not always be known. Cervical incompetence is usually diagnosed with a transvaginal ultrasound, which can show if the cervix is dilated or has shortened. The diagnosis could potentially be confirmed with a biopsy. Treatment for cervical incompetence typically involves bed rest and/or frequent monitoring of the pregnancy. In some cases, a cerclage (a stitch) may be placed around the cervix to hold it closed.

Question 34:

Answer:
C.Improve.

EXPLANATION: Migraine headaches are a common type of headache that can occur during pregnancy. Hannah, who is 14 weeks pregnant, has a previous history of migraines. During pregnancy, her symptoms of migraines are likely to improve. This is because the increased hormones during pregnancy can help to reduce the frequency and severity of migraines. Additionally, pregnancy can help to reduce the stress and anxiety that can trigger migraines. If Hannah is experiencing migraines during her pregnancy, she should talk to her doctor about ways to manage her symptoms.

Question 35:
Answer:
D.All of the above

EXPLANATION: Fetal macrosomia is defined as a birth weight ≥4,000 grams (8 pounds, 13 ounces) or ≥4,500 grams (9 pounds, 15 ounces) for infants born at ≥37 weeks gestation. There are many potential causes of fetal macrosomia, including maternal diabetes, genetic factors, and fetal overgrowth disorders. Maternal diabetes is the most common cause of fetal macrosomia, accounting for 60-70% of cases.1,2 Women with diabetes have high levels of glucose in their blood, which crosses the placenta and causes the fetus to grow larger than normal. Maternal diabetes can be controlled with diet, exercise, and medication, but if it is not well-controlled, it can lead to serious complications for both the mother and the baby. Obesity and overdue pregnancy also play a role in fetal macrosomia.

Question 36:

Answer:
C.37.

EXPLANATION: Preterm is a condition where contractions occur anywhere from 2 to 4 weeks before the baby is to be born. If a mother delivers preterm, it is important to seek medical attention right away as the baby may need special care. Preterm infants are at risk for a number of problems, including respiratory distress, jaundice, and infection. In some cases, preterm infants may also experience developmental delays.

Question 37:

Answer :

A. deep venous thrombosis (DVT)

Explanation : When a woman delivers a baby, her body expels the blood and tissue that built up in her uterus during pregnancy. This is called lochia, and it can last for up to six weeks after delivery. In some cases, women may experience blood clots in their lochia. These clots can range in size from small to golf ball-sized. It is unlikely that Sharon's deep venous thrombosis (DVT) is the cause of her golf ball-sized blood clots in her lochia. DVT is a clot that forms in a deep vein, usually in the leg. It is usually the result of prolonged immobility, such as after surgery. Sharon's blood clots are more likely to be caused by another condition, such as a uterine infection or a postpartum hemorrhage.

Question 38

Answer:

C. Early.

Explanation: When a baby is born, they are typically born with a rooting reflex. This reflex is when the baby's mouth opens and they turn its head to the side in order to find something to suck on. This reflex is what helps the baby to latch onto the breast and start nursing. The rooting reflex typically goes away after the baby is a few weeks old and is no longer needing to breastfeed.

Question 39:

Answer: C.Active sleep

EXPLANATION: Newborns are in a state of active sleep when they are startled awake by sudden noises. Their bodies twitch and their eyes move rapidly beneath closed lids. This is a normal part of the sleep cycle for babies and is nothing to worry about.

Question 40:

Answer:

A. Complete bed rest.

Explanation: Complete bed rest is not an ideal intervention for preventing DVT. The best interventions for preventing a DVT are those that encourage the patient to move around, such as walking and leg exercises. Complete bed rest can actually increase the risk of a DVT because it allows the blood to pool in the veins, which can lead to clot formation.

Question 41

Answer:

D. Estrogen

EXPLANATION: Lactation suppression is the medical term for when a woman stops producing milk. This can happen for a variety of reasons, including weaning, pregnancy loss, or simply because a woman no longer wants to breastfeed. There are a few different methods of lactation suppression, but the most common is to use medication. There are a few different types of medication that can be used to suppress lactation. These include: - Estrogen: Estrogen is a hormone that is known to decrease milk production. It can be consumed as a tablet, a patch, or a gel.- Progestin: Progestin is another hormone that can be used to suppress lactation. It works by fooling the body into thinking that it is pregnant, which decreases milk production. Progestin can be taken in the form of a pill or injection.- Tricyclic antidepressants: Tricyclic antidepressants are a type of medication that is typically used to treat depression. However, they can also be used to suppress lactation.

Question 42:
Answer: B. Deficiency of vitamin K

EXPLANATION: Hemorrhagic disease of the newborn (HDN) is a type of bleeding disorder that can occur in newborns. The disorder is caused by a deficiency of the blood clotting factor vitamin K. HDN can be mild, causing only a small amount of bleeding, or it can be severe, leading to life-threatening bleeding. HDN is most often seen in newborns who are born to mothers who are Rh-negative (the mother's blood does not have the protein that is needed to make the red blood cells clot). When an Rh-negative mother has a baby who is Rh-positive (the baby's blood has the protein that is needed to make the red blood cells clot), Antibodies made by the mother's body could target the baby's red blood cells. These antibodies can cause HDN. HDN can also be caused by a deficiency of vitamin K. The blood must have vitamin K to clot. If a baby does not get enough vitamin K, the blood may not clot properly, and the baby may bleed.

Question 43

Answer:

A. Genetically.

Explanation: Cystic fibrosis is an inherited disorder. This condition damages the lungs, digestive system, and other organs in the body. It affects the cells producing mucus, sweat, and digestive juices. These fluids are normally thin and slippery. Genetically, this disease can be transferred from the mother to the infant.

Question 44:
Answer: C. Antibiotics

EXPLANATION: There are a number of interventions that might help a postpartum patient who has hemorrhoid discomfort, but antibiotics would not be considered one of them. Hemorrhoids are common during pregnancy and the postpartum period and can be a source of considerable discomfort. While they typically resolve on their own, there are a number of things that can be done to help ease the symptoms in the meantime. Ice packs or cold compresses can help to relieve pain and swelling. Topical ointments, creams, or gels can also be helpful, although it is important to avoid those that contain steroids or other ingredients that could potentially be harmful to a nursing mother. Increasing fluid intake and dietary fiber can help to soften the stool and reduce constipation, which can aggravate hemorrhoids. Some people find relief from anal rubbing with a Witch Hazel pad or pad soaked in remedies like Aloe Vera. Sitz baths, in which the affected area is soaked in warm water for 10-15 minutes several times a day, can also be soothing.

Question 45:

Answer:
B. Hemorrhage.

Explanation: When someone suffers a traumatic injury and then dies, the immediate cause of death is typically hemorrhage or uncontrolled bleeding. This can occur both internally, where bleeding occurs within the body cavities, or externally, where blood loss is obvious and severe. In the case of an internal bleed, the patient may lose consciousness and go into shock due to low blood pressure. If the bleeding is not quickly controlled, death will follow. External bleeds are usually more obvious and apparent and can be controlled with direct pressure and tourniquets if necessary. However, if the bleed is not quickly controlled, death will follow. In either case, the cause of death is ultimately hemorrhage. Once bleeding begins, it is very difficult to stop, and death will occur if the patient loses too much blood.

Question 46:

Answer :
C. Diastasis recti abdominis

Explanation: Diastasis recti abdominis is a condition that can occur during pregnancy when the abdominal muscles separate. This can cause pain and discomfort, as well as other symptoms. During pregnancy, the abdominal muscles stretch and loosen to accommodate the growing uterus. This can cause the muscles to separate, which can lead to pain and discomfort. In some cases, the separation may be severe enough to cause hernias.

Question 47:

Answer:
B.Rectally

EXPLANATION: There are a few different ways to administer misoprostol for postpartum bleeding, but the most common and considered correct route is rectally. Misoprostol is a synthetic prostaglandin that is used to help expel the placenta, help contract the uterus, and control heavy bleeding after childbirth. When given rectally, it is slowly absorbed through the tissue lining the rectum and into the bloodstream, where it then travels to the uterus and helps to contract it. This is the most effective way to administer misoprostol for postpartum bleeding because it allows the drug to directly stimulate the uterine muscles and helps to control the bleeding more quickly. Other ways to administer misoprostol include vaginally or orally. However, these methods are not as effective because the drug is not as concentrated in the area where it needs to be. When given vaginally, misoprostol is absorbed through the vaginal tissue and into the bloodstream, but it takes longer for it to reach the uterus and start working.

Question 48:

Answer:
A. Periodic changes.

Explanations: Decelerations or accelerations in the fetal heart rate may correspond to periodic changes in the strength or duration of uterine contractions, known as periodic changes. These changes can be caused by a variety of factors, including the mother's position, the baby's position, the mother's level of activity, and the amount of amniotic fluid around the baby. Although periodic changes are usually harmless, they can sometimes be a sign of a problem, such as fetal distress. If you're concerned about periodic changes, talk to your doctor or midwife.

Question 49:

·

Answer:

B. Bottle feeding. .

EXPLANATION: Involution, the process by which the uterus returns to its nonpregnant state, is improved by many factors. These include good nutrition, adequate rest, and avoidance of smoking and alcohol. On the other hand, bottle feeding can interfere with involution. Bottle feeding, also known as formula feeding, can reduce the amount of oxytocin that is released. Oxytocin is a hormone that helps the uterus contract and return to its nonpregnant state. Therefore, less oxytocin can mean slower involution. Additionally, bottle feeding can cause breast engorgement, which can also interfere with the involution process. It is important to note that while bottle feeding can interfere with involution, it is not the only factor that can do so. Poor nutrition, inadequate rest, and smoking or drinking alcohol can also slow down involution. Therefore, it is best to avoid all of these things if you want to optimize the involution process.

Question 50:

Answer :

B. Low level placenta previa.

Explanation: Low-level placenta previa is when the placenta partially or completely covers the cervix. This can happen during the early stages of labor when the contractions cause the cervix to dilate and the placenta to move out of the way. However, in some cases, the placenta doesn't move out of the way, which can cause the cervix to tear.

Question 51:

Answer :

A. Due to space occupancy by the fetuses there is over-distension of the uterus triggering early labor

Explanation : When it comes to twins, triplets, and even quintuplets, premature birth is often a concern. This is due to space occupancy by the fetuses there is over-distension of the uterus triggering early labor. Multiple births are often associated with a lower birth weight, which can increase the risk of complications. Additionally, multiple births are often associated with a shorter gestation period, which can also increase the risk of complications.

Question 52:
answer) Option
D.   both B and C

Explanation: There are three types of abruptio placenta: marginal, partial, and complete. Marginal abruptio placenta is when the separation occurs at the edge of the placenta and usually does not cause vaginal bleeding. Partial abruptio placenta is when the separation occurs in the middle of the placenta and can cause vaginal bleeding. Complete abruptio placenta is when the separation occurs throughout the entirety of the placenta and can cause vaginal bleeding. While all three types of abruptio placenta can cause vaginal bleeding, it is more likely with partial and complete abruptio placenta.

Question 53:
Answer:
A.Diabetes mellitus
EXPLANATION: Disseminated intravascular coagulation (DIC) is a disorder in which the blood clotting process is activated throughout the body. This can lead to serious problems, such as bleeding and organ damage. DIC most often occurs as a complication of another condition, such as cancer, sepsis (a potentially life-threatening condition caused by infection), or pregnancy. It can also be caused by certain medications or medical procedures. DIC can be a life-threatening condition. If you have symptoms of DIC, seek medical attention immediately. The symptoms of DIC vary depending on how severe the condition is. They may include: • Easy bruising • Skin Rash • Fatigue • Nausea and vomiting • Abdominal pain • Shortness of breath • Pale skin • Cold hands and feet • Lightheadedness or dizziness • Confusion • seizures

Question 54

Answer:
B. Dizziness.
Explanation: The bacteria Chlamydia trachomatis is the source of the sexually transmitted infection (STI) known as chlamydia. It is the most prevalent STI in the United States and can infect both men and women. Most commonly, unprotected vaginal, anal, or oral sex is how chlamydia is transmitted. During childbirth, it can also be passed from an infected mother to her infant. Symptoms of chlamydia may include: -- Watery or white discharge from the vagina or penis -Painful urination -Rectal pain, bleeding, or discharge - Swollen or painful testicles Most people with chlamydia do not have any symptoms. This is why it is important to get tested for STIs regularly, even if you feel healthy and have no symptoms. If chlamydia is not treated, it can lead to serious health problems, such as infertility, pelvic inflammatory disease, and ectopic pregnancy. Dizziness is not a symptom of chlamydia.

Question 55:
Answer: Option
D)over cooked meat causing denaturation of muscle
Explanation: Toxoplasmosis caused by T.gondii is a disease that can be transmitted by many different means. One of the most common ways it is spread is through contact with infected animals, including cats. It can also be spread through contaminated food or water, or from mother to child during pregnancy. Toxoplasmosis is typically a benign condition with no symptoms.. However, it can be severe in some people, causing problems such as brain damage, blindness, and even death. The best way to prevent toxoplasmosis is to avoid contact with contaminated food, water, or animals. If you are pregnant, be sure to talk to your doctor about ways to avoid toxoplasmosis.

Question 56:
Answer:
C. Every 15 minutes for 1 hour and then every 30 minutes for 2 hours.

Explanation: It is important to check a patient's vital signs post-delivery in order to assess their condition and identify any potential complications. The ideal time or frequency for checking vital signs will vary depending on the type of delivery and the patient's individual condition. For normal delivery, it is generally recommended that vital signs be checked every 15 minutes for the first hour and then every 30 minutes for the next two hours. This allows for close monitoring of the patient in the immediate aftermath of delivery and then a less frequent check-in as the patient stabilizes.

Question 57:
Answer:
C. Drugs that are heavily narcotic

EXPLANATION: Around the world, it is estimated that up to 85% of women experience some form of pain during the postpartum period. This pain can range from mild discomfort to severe pain that interferes with daily activities. There are a variety of methods that can be used to relieve postpartum pain, but heavy narcotics or analgesics are not typically recommended. There are a number of reasons why heavy narcotics or analgesics are not recommended for postpartum pain relief. First, these medications can have side effects that can be harmful to both the mother and the baby. These side effects can include drowsiness, constipation, and respiratory depression. In addition, these medications can interfere with the bonding process between the mother and the baby. There are a number of alternative methods that can be used to relieve postpartum pain. These methods include ice or heat packs, massages, relaxation techniques, and over-the-counter pain medications. In some cases, an epidural may be used to relieve pain.

Question 58:

Answer: D. Intertrigo.
 Intertrigo is a common, superficial fungal infection of the skin that typically occurs in hot, humid weather. It most often affects the folds of skin where two skin surfaces rub together, such as the armpits, groin, between the buttocks, and under the breasts. The skin in these areas is often reddish, raw, and very intense. Baby's skin creases appear to be especially susceptible to this rash. Intertrigo is caused by the overgrowth of yeasts and other fungi that naturally live on the skin. These organisms thrive in warm, moist environments, and can cause an infection when the skin is damaged or irritated. Injury to the skin can occur from friction, moisture, and changes in pH. The most common fungi that cause intertrigo are Candida albicans and Candida Tropicalis. Treatment for intertrigo usually consists of keeping the affected area clean and dry and applying an antifungal cream or powder. In more severe cases, an antifungal pill may be necessary.

Question 59:

Answer:
B. Cerebral palsy.

Explanation: Cerebral palsy is a condition that affects a person's ability to control their muscles. It is caused by damage to the nervous system, which can occur before or after birth. The severity of the condition can vary from person to person, but it can often lead to problems with movement and coordination. The most frequent physical disability in children is cerebral palsy.

Question 60:

answer) Option
D.All of the above
Explanation: A trapped placenta is a placenta that is unable to move downwards into the lower part of the uterus during childbirth. This can happen if the placenta is stuck to the side of the uterus, or if it is attached to the cervix. A trapped placenta can also occur if the umbilical cord is wrapped around the neck of the baby, or if the baby is in a breech (bottom-first) position. If a placenta is trapped, it can cause serious problems for both the mother and the baby. The placenta is responsible for delivering oxygen and nutrients to the baby, and if it is trapped, the baby may not be able to get enough of these vital substances. This can lead to health problems for the baby, including cerebral palsy, mental retardation, and even death. For the mother, a trapped placenta can cause excessive bleeding, which can be life-threatening. Additionally, the placenta may need to be removed surgically, which can be a complicated and risky procedure

Question 61:

Answer: A)variable/ectopic pulse
EXPLANATION: In the case of cervical insufficiency, also known as an incompetent cervix, the main symptom is that the cervix begins to open too early during the pregnancy before the baby is ready to be born. This can lead to premature birth or even miscarriage. However, there are other symptoms that may be seen in cases of cervical insufficiency, including:

-Abnormal vaginal bleeding

-Pelvic pain

-Discharge

-Dilation of the cervix

An ectopic pulse, or an abnormal heartbeat, is not a symptom that is typically seen in cases of cervical insufficiency.

Question 62:
Answer:
B.AFI = 5 cm.

Explanation: To determine the amniotic fluid index (AFI), divide the pregnant uterus into quadrants and then measure the largest vertical pocket of amniotic fluid in each quadrant (measurements are made in centimeters). Add up the largest measurements from each quadrant to get the AFI. The AFI can range from 5-25 cm, with 5-10 cm being considered low and 25 cm or more being considered high. Anything below 5 cm is considered abnormal and warrants further testing. There are several possible causes of low amniotic fluid levels. One is oligohydramnios, which is defined as less than 500 mL of amniotic fluid. This can be caused by things like leakage of fluid from the amniotic sac, decreased production of fluid by the fetus, or increased absorption of fluid by the fetus. Other possible causes include intrauterine growth restriction, premature rupture of membranes, and placental insufficiency. Low amniotic fluid levels can lead to a number of complications.

Question 63:

Answer:
D.1st trimester.
Explanation: While all stages of fetal development are important, the first trimester is when the risk of developing gross abnormalities is the highest. This is because the majority of organs and systems are formed during this time. If there is a problem with the development of any of these structures, it can lead to a birth defect. One of the most common birth defects is a neural tube defect, which occurs when the neural tube, which will become the baby's brain and spinal cord, does not close properly. This can happen if the fetus does not get enough folic acid, a nutrient found in leafy green vegetables, legumes, and fortified foods. Other birth defects can occur if the fetus is exposed to certain substances, such as alcohol, tobacco, or certain medications.

Question 64:

Answer:
A. Breakdown of erythrocytes
EXPLANATION: When a pregnant woman carrying a fetus with a different blood type, the incompatibility between the two can lead to Hemolytic Disease of the Newborn (HDN). This occurs when the mother's antibodies cross the placenta and attack the fetus's red blood cells, causing them to break down. If left untreated, HDN can be fatal. In Jenny's case, her fetus is Rh positive and she is Rh negative. This means that her body will produce antibodies to the Rh factor, which is found on the surface of red blood cells. When these antibodies come into contact with the fetus's red blood cells, they will cause them to break down. There are two types of HDN: mild and severe. Mild HDN is typically treated with a transfusion of Rh-positive red blood cells to the fetus. This helps to increase the fetus's red blood cell count and prevent further destruction of the cells.

Question 65:

Answer:
B. Growth and development of the fetus to survive in the external environment

EXPLANATION: At 28 weeks of pregnancy, fetal development is focused on the growth and development of the fetus to survive in the external environment. The fetus becomes more active and has more energy, and starts to open its eyes and blink. It also develops the ability to feel pain. The bones and muscles continue to grow and strengthen. The lungs also continue to develop, and the amount of amniotic fluid starts to decrease.

Question 66:

Answer:

A. Polyhydramnios

EXPLANATION: Polyhydramnios, also known as hydramnios, is a condition that occurs during pregnancy when there is too much amniotic fluid surrounding the fetus. This excess fluid can cause the mother to experience a variety of symptoms, including shortness of breath, discomfort in the abdomen, and an increased risk of premature labor. Polyhydramnios can also lead to complications during delivery, such as umbilical cord prolapse, and it can increase the risk of a cesarean section. The exact cause of polyhydramnios is often unknown, but it can be due to a leak in the amniotic sac, multiple fetuses (such as twins or triplets), genetic disorders, or maternal diabetes. In some cases, polyhydramnios may resolve on their own without any treatment. However, if the condition is severe or persists, doctors may recommend medications to reduce the amount of amniotic fluid, or they may induce labor.

Question 67:

answer) Option

C.Via point of separation of the placenta

Explanation: When a woman goes into labor, her body starts to push the baby and the placenta out of the uterus. The placenta is attached to the uterus by the umbilical cord, and as it starts to come out, the cord stretches and can rupture. This rupture can cause the amniotic fluid to enter maternal circulation. The amniotic fluid is a clear, slightly yellowish fluid that surrounds the baby in the uterus. It is made up of water, electrolytes, and other substances. The fluid helps to protect the baby from shocks, jolts, and infection. It also provides a cushion for the baby to move around. When the cord ruptures, the amniotic fluid can enter maternal circulation through the point of rupture. This may take place prior to, during, or following childbirth. This may take place prior to, during, or following childbirth. This may take place prior to, during, or following childbirth. This may take place prior to, during, or following childbirth.. If it happens before birth, it is called a pre-labor rupture of membranes (PROM). If it happens during the birth, it is called an intrapartum rupture of membranes (IRA).

Question 68:

Answer:

A. Before 20 weeks of pregnancy.

Explanation When a woman experiences a miscarriage also called a spontaneous abortion, it typically occurs before 20 weeks of pregnancy. While the exact cause is not always known, there are several possible explanations, including - Hormonal imbalances: This can cause the uterine lining to break down, making it difficult for the embryo to implant and thrive. - Anatomical problems: If the uterus is abnormally shaped or there are other issues with the reproductive organs, it can make it difficult for the embryo to implant properly. - Infection: An infection in the uterus can cause the tissue to break down, leading to a miscarriage. - Chromosomal abnormalities: If the embryo has abnormal chromosomes, it is often unable to develop properly and will miscarry. If you think you may be at risk for miscarrying, it is important to talk to your doctor so that they can help you manage your risk factors.

Question 69:
answer: Option
B) Hepatic rupture

Explanation: In this case, it is suspected that Kate has suffered a hepatic rupture. This is a serious condition that can occur when the liver is damaged, typically due to a traumatic injury. If not treated promptly, it can lead to severe bleeding and death. Treatment for a hepatic rupture typically involves surgery to repair the damage. In Kate's case, she will likely need to have a C-section to deliver her baby. She will also need close monitoring during her recovery.

Question 70:
.

Answer: Watch for uterine atony.
Explanation: At the latent stage of labor, the nurse's primary responsibility is to monitor the mother and baby for signs of distress. The nurse should also be alert for any changes in the mother's contractions or the baby's heart rate. If any problems are detected, the nurse should notify the doctor or midwife immediately. Watching for uterine atony is not a key responsibility of the nurse at the latent stage of labor.

Question 71:

Answer :
B. The fetal and placental membranes

Explanation The placental and fetal membranes are the primary means of heat dissipation for the fetus. The fetal membrane is a thin layer of tissue that covers the fetus and separates it from the amniotic fluid in the womb. The placental membrane is a thicker layer of tissue that attaches the fetus to the uterine wall. Both membranes are permeable to heat, allowing the fetus to regulate its own body temperature. The fetal and placental membranes are also the primary means of exchanging nutrients and wastes between the fetus and the mother. The maternal blood supply passes through the placental membrane, providing the fetus with oxygen and nutrients. The fetal blood supply passes through the fetal membrane, returning oxygen and nutrient-depleted blood to the mother. Waste products from the fetus are also transferred through the fetal membrane to the mother, where they are eliminated. Maternal and fetal circulation are intimately linked, and the placental and fetal membranes play a crucial role in this relationship. The maternal blood supply provides the fetus with the oxygen and nutrients it needs to grow and develop.

Question 72:

Answer:

B. 5-10%

Explanation: A newborn can afford to lose 5-10% of their body weight in the first week of life without any significant adverse consequences. This is because a newborn's body is still developing and thus has a greater capacity for weight loss than an adult. Additionally, a newborn has a higher percentage of body water than an adult, which helps to offset any weight loss. There are a number of reasons why a newborn may lose weight in the first week of life. One common reason is simply due to the loss of residual meconium, which is the first stool a newborn passes. Meconium is typically dark and tarry in appearance and can weigh up to 5% of a newborn's body weight. Another common reason for weight loss in newborns is due to insufficient intake of calories. This can be due to a number of reasons, such as poor latch, inability to suck, or difficulty swallowing. Additionally, newborns have a relatively small stomach capacity, meaning they need to eat more frequently than adults.

Question 73:

Answer: B. Weight

Explanation Lochia is the vaginal discharge that a woman experiences after giving birth. It is made up of blood, mucus, and tissue from the lining of the uterus. Lochia usually starts out heavy and bright red, but it gradually decreases in amount and changes to a lighter pink or brown over the course of several weeks Lochia shouldn't smell bad at all. There are several factors that a nurse should examine when assessing a patient's lochia. These include the color, amount, and odor of the discharge. However, weight is not a factor that should be considered.

Question 74:

Answer:

A. Ultrasound is used to measure the fetal heart rate. Contractions are measured using pressure sensor.

EXPLANATION: Contractions are measured using a pressure sensor. External electronic fetal monitoring (EFM) is a method for monitoring fetal heart rate (FHR) and uterine contractions during labor. It generally consists of two parts: an ultrasound transducer placed on the mother's abdomen to measure the FHR, and a tocodynamometer (pressure sensor) placed on the mother's abdomen or vagina to measure the strength and frequency of contractions. There are two types of EFM: intermittent and continuous. Intermittent EFM is when the monitors are attached and turned on for only a few minutes at a time, typically every 15-30 minutes. This allows the mother to move around and change positions more easily. Continuous EFM is when the monitors are attached and turned on continuously. This provides a more constant and uninterrupted monitoring of the FHR and contractions but can be more uncomfortable for the mother.

Question 75:
Answer:

D. Congenital abnormalities

EXPLANATION: A congenital abnormality is an anomaly that is present at birth. This can be a physical defect, such as a heart defect, or a mental disability, such as Down Syndrome. Congenital abnormalities are one of the leading causes of newborn mortality. There are many different types of congenital abnormalities, and the odds of a baby being born with one are relatively low. However, certain factors can increase the risk. These include: - Advanced maternal age - Exposure to certain drugs or infections during pregnancy - Genetic disorders . Congenital abnormalities can often be detected before birth through prenatal testing. This can allow parents to make informed decisions about the pregnancy and delivery. In some cases, corrective surgery can be performed before or after birth.

Question 76:

Answer:

A.To measure the fetal well-being and fetal oxygen supply

EXPLANATION: Fetal Kick Count is defined as the number of times a pregnant woman feels her baby move over a period of two hours. This is generally done in the later stages of pregnancy, typically after 28 weeks. The fetal kick count is important in order to measure the fetal well-being and fetal oxygen supply. The fetal heart rate is an important indicator of fetal health, and the fetal kick count can help to assess this. A fetus's heart beats normally between 120 and 160 times per minute. A lower heart rate may indicate that the fetus is not getting enough oxygen, and a higher heart rate may indicate that the fetus is under stress. The fetal kick count can also help to assess whether the fetus is getting enough oxygen by counting the number of times the fetus moves. A normal fetal movement should occur at least 10 times in a two-hour period. A lower number of fetal movements may indicate that the fetus is not getting enough oxygen, and a higher number of fetal movements may indicate that the fetus is under stress.

Question 77
Answer :

C. his bone marrow does not produce enough blood cells

Explanation: When a baby is born, its bone marrow begins to produce blood cells. These blood cells are essential for carrying oxygen and other nutrients to the cells in the body. Without enough blood cells, the body cannot function properly. In Stacy's son's case, his bone marrow does not produce enough blood cells. This can be a result of many different things, such as a genetic condition, a viral infection, or a problem with the bone marrow itself. Whatever the cause, it is important to get treatment for this condition as soon as possible. If not treated, Stacy's son's condition will only get worse. He will become increasingly pale and will have difficulty breathing. He may also develop other problems, such as an infection or bleeding. If not treated, this condition can be fatal. Fortunately, there are treatments available that can help Stacy's son. One treatment option is a blood transfusion, which can help to increase the level of blood cells in the body. Another option is medication, which can help to stimulate the bone marrow to produce more blood cells.

Question 78

Answer :

C. Miliria (prickly heat)

Explanation: When a newborn is unable to regulate their body heat, they are at risk for a condition called miliria. Miliria is a skin condition that presents as a rash of tiny, red bumps. The lumps can hurt and are frequently irritating. In some cases, the bumps may blister. Miliria is caused by exposure to extreme heat. Newborns are particularly vulnerable to this condition because their skin is very thin and their sweat glands are not fully developed. When exposed to extreme heat, the sweat glands can become blocked, causing the sweat to build up under the skin. This can lead to inflammation and the formation of the bumps. Miliria is most common in hot, humid weather. However, it can also occur in dry heat. It is more likely to occur if a newborn is overdressed or if they are in a car seat or stroller that is in direct sunlight. If your newborn has miliria, it is important to keep them cool and comfortable.

Question 79:

answer) Option c)3

Explanation: The number of phases seen in amniotic fluid embolism is: 1) The initial phase, where the woman may experience a sudden onset of shortness of breath and chest pain. 2) The second phase, where the woman's blood pressure may drop and she may go into cardiac arrest. 3) The third and final phase, where the woman may suffer from seizures and organ failure.

Question 80

Answer :

C. 40-60 cycles per minute

Explanation: When a baby is born, its respiration rate is usually between 40 and 60 cycles per minute. This rate may differ slightly depending on the baby's age, weight, and health status. Respiration rates can also be affected by environmental factors such as temperature and humidity. In general, however, a respiration rate of 40-60 cycles per minute is considered normal for a newborn. A newborn's respiration rate is usually faster than an adult's respiration rate. This is because a newborn's body is still adjusting to life outside of the womb. Their bodies are working hard to regulate their temperature, breathing, and heart rate. As a result, a newborn's respiration rate may be higher than normal for the first few days or weeks of life. It is important to monitor a newborn's respiration rate and seek medical attention if their rate is consistently above 60 cycles per minute.

Question 81:

Answer :

D. Inadequate development of infant's respiratory center

Explanation: Anatomically, the respiratory center is located in the medulla oblongata and the pons. The medulla oblongata contains the inspiratory neurons while the expiratory neurons are located in the pons. Both the inspiratory and expiratory neurons are innervated by the vagus nerve (cranial nerve X). The respiratory center controls the rate and depth of breathing. The rate of breathing is determined by the frequency of firing of the inspiratory neurons while the depth of breathing is determined by the amplitude of the signal from the inspiratory neurons. In a premature baby, the respiratory center may not be fully developed. This can lead to a condition called apnea, which is defined as a period of time where there is no breathing. Apnea can be caused by a variety of factors, including a lack of stimulus to the respiratory center (such as a low blood oxygen level), a build-up of carbon dioxide in the blood, or a problem with the respiratory center itself.

Question 82:

Answer:

C. Late cue If the infant turns red and cries, they would be at the late cue level of readiness to nurse. This is because they are showing signs of hunger and need, but they are not yet latched on or actively sucking. The mother will need to help the infant latch on and begin nursing.

Question 83:
Answer:

D. effective removal of milk from the breast

EXPLANATION: The most important factor for the mother to maintain lactation is the effective removal of milk from the breast. If milk is not effectively removed from the breast, the mother's body will not receive the signal to continue producing milk. Additionally, milk that is not removed from the breast can lead to engorgement, which can be painful and lead to infection.

Question 84:

Answer:

A.Food addiction/Milk Addiction

Explanation There are a number of risks associated with obesity, but food addiction or milk addiction is not one of them. Obesity is a risk factor for a number of conditions, including heart disease.

Question 85:
Answer:
B. Maternal Role Attainment
Explanation: Maternal role attainment is a process through which mothers learn and develop the skills and knowledge necessary to effectively care for their children. The process is often divided into three stages: learning, performance, and mastery.

Question 86:

Answer:
A.125 to 200 milliunits/minute
EXPLANATION: Oxytocin is a hormone that is produced naturally in the body. It is released from the pituitary gland and acts on the uterus to help control muscle contractions during childbirth. Oxytocin is also sometimes given intravenously (IV) to help control postpartum bleeding. The recommended dose of oxytocin for IV use is 125 to 200 milliunits/minute. This dose is typically given as a continuous infusion over a period of several hours. The total amount of oxytocin given will depend on the individual situation and how much bleeding is present.

Question 87:
Answer:
B. Every 15 minutes
EXPLANATION: Every 15 minutes, a healthcare professional will auscultate, or listen to, the fetal heart rate, on a woman who is in the second stage of labor. This is to make sure that the fetus is not experiencing any distress and is overall well-being. If the fetal heart rate is found to be abnormal, or if the woman is experiencing any other complications, the Healthcare provider may order more frequent monitoring.

Question 88:

Answer:
D.All of the above
EXPLANATION: Chorioamnionitis is an infection of the fetal membrane and chorion, the outermost layer of the placenta. It is a rare but potentially serious complication of pregnancy that can lead to preterm labor and delivery, as well as sepsis and death. The most common symptoms of chorioamnionitis are fever, uterine tenderness, and fetal tachycardia. Other signs and symptoms may include leukocytosis, maternal tachycardia, and preterm rupture of membranes.
The most common cause of chorioamnionitis is bacteria ascending from the mother's vagina or cervix into the uterus. This can happen due to several different factors, including ruptured membranes, vaginal infections, sexually transmitted infections, or urinary tract infections. Additionally, chorioamnionitis can occur in pregnancies where the mothers have underlying medical conditions that make them more susceptible to infection, such as diabetes or immunodeficiency.

Question 89:

Answer :
A. raised heart rate
Explanation: Raised heart rate is not a sign of deep vein thrombosis (DVT) in a bedridden patient. The lower limbs and abdomen should be examined for DVT. A deep vein thrombus, or DVT, develops most frequently in the leg. Symptoms of DVT include swelling, pain, and redness in the affected limb. If the clot dislodges, it may move to the lungs and result in a potentially fatal pulmonary embolism.

Question 90:

Answer :
C. club foot
Explanation: A clubfoot is a congenital deformity in which the foot is twisted out of shape or position. The most common form of clubfoot is where the foot is turned inwards and downwards at the ankle. This can cause the individual to walk on the outer edge of the foot or on their toes. Clubfoot is thought to be caused by a combination of genetic and environmental factors. It is more common in males than females, with a ratio of around 2:1. It is also more common in certain ethnic groups, such as Native Americans, Asians, and Pacific Islanders.

Question 91

Answer:
A. Weight loss of at least 30 pounds.
Explanation: Uterine involution is the process by which the uterus shrinks back to its non-pregnant size and shape following childbirth. This process begins immediately after delivery and is complete by around six weeks postpartum. weight loss of at least 30 pounds is not involved in uterine involution. involution involves three main changes: 1. The decrease in size of the uterine cavity 2. The reduction in thickness of the uterine walls 3. The return of the uterine blood vessels to their pre-pregnancy state The first two changes are essential for the third to occur. The reduction in the size of the uterine cavity is brought about by the muscular contraction of the uterine walls.

Question 92:

Answer:
A. 9-18 months of age.
Explanation: A newborn infant's anterior fontanelle is a diamond-shaped soft spot located on the top of the head where the bones of the skull have not yet completely joined. This soft spot allows the infant's head to change shape during birth and permits small amounts of movement between the bones of the skull, which helps the brain to grow. The anterior fontanelle usually closes by 9-18 months of age as the bones of the skull fuse together. During the first few months of life, the fontanelles permit slight movements of the skull bones, which helps the brain to grow.

Question 93:

Answer:
A. Teratogens.
Explanation: A chemical that can result in birth abnormalities is called a teratogen. The effects of a teratogen can be different depending on the timing of exposure during pregnancy. If a pregnant woman is exposed to a teratogen during the first trimester, when the baby's organs are developing, it is more likely to cause a birth defect than if she is exposed during the second trimester, when the baby's bones and muscles are developing. There are many different types of teratogens, including medications, environmental toxins, and infections. Some common examples of teratogens are alcohol, mercury, lead, certain viruses, and certain medications.

Question 94:
Answer : D)firm and flat

Explanation:The cranial sutures are sites of approximation of cranial bones. Since these are opposed by bones their consistency is firm and flat. The meeting point of the sutures is at the level of fontanelles. infants skull is made up of many bones that are connected together by sutures. The sutures allow for movement of the bones during birth and growth. As the infant grows, the sutures begin to fuse and the bones become rigid. The bones of the skull are thick and the sutures are shallow. This makes it difficult to feel the sutures with your fingers. However, if you place your hand on the infant's head and move your fingers along the suture lines, you should be able to feel a slight indentation.

Question 95:

Answer :
C. Warm blankets
Explanation: For Casey, a pregnant mother who recently delivered, one intervention that may be helpful is the use of warm blankets. This is because many new mothers experience a drop in body temperature after giving birth, which can contribute to feelings of fatigue and flu-like symptoms. By using warm blankets, Casey can help to regulate her body temperature and hopefully reduce some of these discomforting side effects. In addition to warm blankets, other interventions that may be helpful for Casey include 1. Rest – it is important for Casey to get as much rest as possible, both during the day and at night. This will help her to physically recover from childbirth and also to deal with the inevitable sleep deprivation that comes with caring for a newborn.

Question 96

Answer:
B. Fertilization age.

Explanation: Fertilization takes place when the sperm penetrates the egg and the egg is fertilized. The age of the embryo is then calculated from the date of the last menstrual period (LMP). The LMP is used as a starting point because it is easy to calculate, but it is only an estimate of when ovulation and fertilization occurred. In a typical 28-day cycle, ovulation occurs around day 14, so the fertilization age would be 14 days. However, not all women have a 28-day cycle, so the fertilization age may be different. The fertilization age is important because it is used to calculate the due date. The due date is calculated by adding 40 weeks (280 days) to the LMP. This gives an estimate of when the baby will be born. However, it is just an estimate, and most babies are born within two weeks of the due date. The fertilization age is also used to calculate the gestational age.

Question 97:
Answer:
A.   2 months or even before.
    EXPLANATION: When an infant is born, the skull bones have not yet fused together. There are several areas where the skull bones remain unfused, and these are known as fontanelles. The two largest fontanelles are the anterior fontanelle, located at the front of the head, and the posterior fontanelle, located at the back of the head. The posterior fontanelle typically closes at 2 months of age, or even before. This is because the bones of the skull begin to fuse together at this age. However, the anterior fontanelle usually remains open for longer, and can take up to 18 months to close. The fontanelles allow for the expansion of the skull during the birth process and the early months of life. They also allow the skull to absorb impact in the case of a fall or other trauma. The posterior fontanelle is typically the last of the fontanelles to close.

Question 98:

Answer: D. O negative (O-).
Explanation   When a baby is born with blood group B negative, it means that they have inherited a blood type that is not typically found in nature. This can happen for a number of reasons, but it usually happens when the father and mother have different blood types. In this case, the mother would likely be blood type O negative. The reason that this is a problem is because when a baby has a blood type that is not compatible with their mother's, it can cause a condition called hemolytic jaundice. This is a condition where the baby's red blood cells are destroyed at a faster rate than they can be replaced.

Question 99:

Answer:
A. Decreases the RBC of the baby

Explanation: There are many potential effects of alcohol consumption during pregnancy, but decreasing the red blood cells (RBC) of the baby is not one of them. RBCs are responsible for carrying oxygen throughout the body, so if their levels are decreased, it could lead to serious health problems for the baby. Additionally, alcohol consumption during pregnancy has been linked to an increased risk of miscarriage, preterm labor, and stillbirth. It is also important to note that alcohol breaks down more slowly in the developing baby than in the mother, so the baby is exposed to its effects for longer periods of time. For these reasons, it is recommended that pregnant women abstain from alcohol completely to ensure the health of their babies.

Question 100:

answer) Option
D. It is related to a decrease in uterine contractions

Explanation: In labor, tachysystole refers to excessive contractions.
This condition has been found to be associated with decelerations in fetal heart rate, and is therefore relevant not only to the mother's comfort but to the baby's well-being as well.

Question 101:

Answer:
A. Tachypnea.
Explanation: A newborn in the maternity ward is seen to have 60 breaths per minute. This is called tachypnea and is a normal finding in newborns. A respiratory rate of more than 60 breaths per minute is referred to as tachypnea. It is a common finding in newborns and is usually nothing to worry about. However, if tachypnea is associated with other symptoms such as difficulty breathing, blue lips or skin, or increased work of breathing, it may be a sign of a serious problem and medical attention should be sought.

Question 102:

Answer:
C.Metritis.
Explanation: Metritis is a uterine infection that can occur after a woman gives birth. It can also occur after a miscarriage or an abortion. Metritis can cause a woman to feel sick and can lead to problems such as fever, pain, and a bad smell coming from the vagina. If not treated, metritis can cause long-term problems such as infertility.

Question 103:

answer) Option
B) The statement is correct, the fertilized ovum has 46 chromosome

Explanation: A fertilized ovum, or egg, typically contains 23 chromosomes from the mother and 23 from the father. This gives the egg a total of 46 chromosomes. This is the diploid number and is found in most of the cells of the human body. The only cells that have a different number of chromosomes are the sex cells, or gametes, which have half the number of chromosomes as the other cells in the body. This is because gametes are formed through a process called meiosis, which halves the number of chromosomes.

Question 104:

Answer:
A. Identified during the blood work of 1st trimester.
Explanation: Placenta accreta is a condition that occurs when the placenta grows too deeply into the uterine wall. This can occur for a number of reasons, including previous scar tissue from a C-section or other uterine surgery. Placenta accreta can also be caused by a rare condition called basal cell Nevus syndrome. This condition is characterized by the overgrowth of the placenta, and can lead to a number of complications during pregnancy, including hemorrhage, premature birth, and even death. While the exact symptoms of placenta accreta can vary depending on the severity of the condition, there are some common symptoms that are associated with this condition. These symptoms can include bleeding during pregnancy, abnormal uterine bleeding, and abdominal pain. In some cases, placenta accreta can also lead to the development of placenta previa, which is a condition where the placenta covers the cervix. This can be a very dangerous complication, as it can lead to major bleeding during childbirth.

Question 105

Answer:
C. Both A and B.
Explanation: When the umbilical cord becomes prolapsed, the baby is no longer receiving oxygen and nutrients from the placenta. This can cause the baby to become distressed and exhibit signs of hypoxia (low oxygen levels). The baby's heart rate will usually become rapid and irregular, and the baby may become limp and unresponsive. In severe cases, the baby may go into cardiac arrest. Also the mother may feel the chord.

Question 106

Answer: A.Cardiorespiratory
EXPLANATION: As a baby is born, they transition from intrauterine (inside the mother) to extrauterine (outside the womb). During this time, there are multiple changes that occur in the cardiorespiratory system. The main change is that the baby starts to breathe on their own. Until this point, they have been getting oxygen from the placenta via the umbilical cord. When they take their first breath, they start to inhale oxygen and exhale carbon dioxide. This exchange of gases continues throughout their life. The other main change that occurs is in the heart. When the baby is in the womb, the heart is located on the right side of the body. This is because the lungs are not yet developed and so the heart doesn't need to pump blood to them. Once the baby is born, the heart moves to the left side of the body and starts to pump blood to the lungs. These are just some of the changes that occur in the cardiorespiratory system when a baby is born.

Question 107:

answer: Option
B)hypovolemic shock

Explanation The most common complication associated with hepatic rupture is a hypovolemic shock. This occurs when the liver is not able to produce enough blood to circulate throughout the body. The liver is responsible for making sure that blood sugar levels are regulated and that the blood clotting process happens properly. When the liver is not functioning properly, these functions are not able to happen, and the result is a hypovolemic shock. Symptoms of hypovolemic shock include low blood pressure, dizziness, lightheadedness, and fainting. If not treated immediately, hypovolemic shock can lead to death. Treatment for hypovolemic shock includes restoring the body's fluids and electrolytes. This can be done through IV fluids and intravascular volume expansion.

Question 108:

Answer:
A. Non-Stress Test.

Explanation: An NST, or non-stress test, is a type of fetal monitoring that is used to assess the well-being of a baby during pregnancy. It is usually done after the woman has reached 24 weeks of gestation, and is considered to be a low-risk procedure. The test involves the use of a fetal monitor to measure the baby's heart rate in response to movements. The heart rate is measured for a period of 20 minutes, and the results are then used to determine if the baby is getting enough oxygen and is developing normally. There are two types of NSTs: the standard NST and the modified NST. The standard NST is the most common type of test, and is used to assess the baby's heart rate in response to movements. The modified NST is used when there are concerns about the baby's heart rate or if the mother has a medical condition that may affect the test results. The NST is a safe and non-invasive way to monitor the well-being of a baby during pregnancy.

Question 109

answer) Option
A)Preeclampsia

Explanation: Preeclampsia is a hypertensive disorder of pregnancy, characterized by high blood pressure and proteinuria, that can occur after 20 weeks of gestation. The most common symptoms include headache, pain in the upper right quadrant, and epigastric pain. Other symptoms can include nausea, vomiting, blurred vision, and edemA. Laboratory findings can include elevated ALP and AST. Preeclampsia is a potentially life-threatening condition that can progress to eclampsia, a severe form of the disorder characterized by seizures. Preeclampsia can also lead to placental abruption, a serious complication in which the placenta abruptly separates from the uterus.

Question 110

Answer:
A. Persistent pulmonary hypertension.

Explanation: ECMO (extracorporeal membrane oxygenation) is used whenever there is a need for long-term oxygenation and/or ventilation support. Examples of indications for ECMO support include, but are not limited to, the following: -Persistent pulmonary hypertension -Severe respiratory failure not responding to conventional medical therapy -Cardiac failure not responding to conventional medical therapy -Severe congenital heart defects ECMO can be used as a bridge to lung transplantation, a bridge to cardiac transplantation, or as a destination therapy. ECMO works by taking blood from the patient and circulating it through an artificial lung (the membrane oxygenator) which adds oxygen to the blood and removes carbon dioxide. The oxygenated blood is then returned to the patient. This process bypasses the patient's natural respiratory system.

Question 111:

Answer :
B. para
Explanation: Para is a medical term used to describe the number of times a woman has carried a pregnancy to full term. In Tina's case, she has carried three pregnancies to full term, which would be considered para 3. Para is generally used in reference to the number of live births a woman has had, but can also be used to describe the number of times a woman has been pregnant, regardless of whether the pregnancy ended in a live birth.

Question 112:
answer : Option
A) stimulation of the vagus nerve (vagal response)
Explanation: Uterine contractions during pregnancy are vital to the health of both the mother and the baby. they help to move the baby into the correct position for birth, and they also help to expel the placenta after the baby is born. early deceleration, which is a decrease in the baby's heart rate, can occur due to uterine contractions. This is caused by the stimulation of the vagus nerve, which is responsible for the regulation of heart rate.

Question 113:

Answer :
B. absence of pyrexia
Explanation: A cesarean section is a type of surgery in which the baby is delivered through an incision in the mother's abdomen. After a cesarean section, it is important for the incision to heal properly to prevent infection. Infection is a common complication of cesarean section and can occur in the mother or the baby. Symptoms of the infection in the mother include fever, redness or swelling at the incision site, and discharge from the incision. Symptoms of the infection in the baby include fever, irritability, and poor feeding. If you are concerned that you or your baby may have an infection, it is important to see a healthcare provider.

Question 114:

Answer:
B.more than 42 weeks of gestation

EXPLANATION: Pregnancy is considered to be post-term when it extends beyond 42 weeks of gestation. This is typically measured from the first day of the woman's last menstrual period (LMP), meaning that post-term pregnancies are those that go beyond 42 weeks from the LMP. In some cases, however, pregnancy may be post-term based on other methods of estimating gestational age, such as ultrasound. There are a number of reasons why a pregnancy may go beyond the 42-week mark. In some cases, it may be due to a delayed or irregular menstrual cycle, making it difficult to pinpoint the exact date of conception.

Question 115:

Answer:

A. Toxemia (Preeclampsia)

EXPLANATION: Lily, a 30-year-old female, is 31 weeks pregnant and is showing symptoms of uncontrolled asthma that may cause several fetal problems, excluding preeclampsia (toxaemia). High blood pressure and protein in the urine are symptoms of the illness known as preeclampsia, which can develop during pregnancy. If left untreated, preeclampsia can lead to serious complications, including eclampsia (seizures), organ damage, and even death. While there is no cure for preeclampsia, early diagnosis and treatment can help manage the condition and reduce the risks to both mother and child.

Question 116:

Answer: A . size and weight of the placenta

Explanation: There are several factors that play a role in the incomplete expulsion of the placenta in a postpartum woman. Firstly, the size and weight of the placenta can play a role. If the placenta is large or heavier than normal, it can be more difficult to expel. Secondly, the position of the placenta can play a role. If the placenta is located in the upper part of the uterus, it can be more difficult to expel. Finally, the tone of the uterus can play a role. If the uterus is not contracting effectively, it can be more difficult to expel the placenta.

Question 117:

Answer:

A.Precipitous

Explanation: A precipitous delivery is one that takes place very rapidly, typically within three hours of the onset of contractions. This can be a very dangerous situation for both the mother and the baby, as there is a higher risk of complications and injuries. The most serious complication is uterine rupture, which can lead to life-threatening hemorrhage. Therefore, it is important for women who think they may be experiencing a precipitous delivery to seek medical help immediately. Once at the hospital, the mother will be closely monitored and may be given medication to help slow down the labor. In some cases, a C-section may be necessary to prevent complications.

Question 118:
Answer :

B. Thermoregulation

Explanation: Brown adipose tissue (BAT) is a type of fat that is found in animals, humans, and other mammals. It is brown due to the presence of mitochondria, which give it its color. BAT is made up of fat cells that are packed together and have many blood vessels running through them. Brown fat tissue is found in the neck, chest, and back. It makes up about 5-10% of the total fat in the body. The main function of BAT is to help the body regulate its temperature. When the body is cold, brown fat cells release a hormone called norepinephrine. Norepinephrine signals the body to burn more calories and produce heat. Brown fat cells are very good at burning calories and producing heat.

Question 119:

Answer :
C. Small ears

Explanation: A genetic disorder called fragile X syndrome results in a variety of developmental issues. The most common features of fragile X syndrome include intellectual disability, behavioral problems such as anxiety and ADHD, and physical features such as large ears, long face, and macrocephaly. Small ears are not a characteristic of fragile X syndrome. One of the most common physical features of fragile X syndrome is large, or protruding, ears. This is due to the changes in the structure of the ear cartilage in individuals with the condition. Other common physical features of fragile X syndrome include a long face, macrocephaly (an enlarged head), and a broad forehead.

Question 120:
answer: Option
C)Chronic hypertension

Explanation: The patient has chronic hypertension if she has a blood pressure above 140/90 mm of hg in her readings prior to pregnancy. This is a condition that can lead to serious complications during pregnancy, so it is important for the patient to be closely monitored by her healthcare provider.

Question 121:
Answer:
C. Low estrogen level in normal pregnancy.

Explanation There are many potential causes for prolonged pregnancy, but one of the most common is a low estrogen level. In a normal pregnancy, estrogen helps to mature the cervix and prepare the uterus for labor. However, if the estrogen level is too low, the cervix may not be able to ripen properly and the uterus may not be able to contract effectively, leading to a prolonged pregnancy. Other potential causes of a prolonged pregnancy include a history of previous prolonged pregnancies, obesity, diabetes, and certain medications.

Question 122:

Answer:
C.Fetal doppler
EXPLANATION: Fetal doppler is a device that is used to listen to the fetal heartbeat. It is not indicated for assessing fetal well-being as it does not provide any information about the fetal heart rate or rhythm.

Question 123:
Answer:
A. After the amniotic sac has ruptured.
Explanation: Internal fetal monitoring (IFM) can only be performed when the amniotic sac has ruptured. This is because the IFM device needs to be inserted through the vagina and cervix into the uterus in order to measure the fetal heart rate (FHR) and uterine contractions. There are two types of IFM: intermittent and continuous. Intermittent IFM is when the FHR and contractions are measured for a set period of time (usually 20 minutes) and then the device is removed. Continuous IFM is when the measurements are taken continuously for the duration of labor. IFM is generally used when there are concerns about the well-being of the fetus, such as when the FHR is not being monitored externally (through a tocodynamometer or Doppler fetal monitor) or when there are concerns about uterine contractions. IFM can also be used for educational purposes, to show the mother and/or father what is happening with their baby during labor.

Question 124:

Answer:
D. Skin breakouts.
Explanation: A skin break out can be an indication of a serious infection, so it is important to examine the post-partum mother's breast for any skin breakouts. While examining the breast, the doctor will look for any redness, swelling, or warmth, which can all be signs of an infection. If an infection is present, the doctor will likely prescribe antibiotics.

Question 125:

Answer :
D. inflammation of Fallopian tubes/ovaries
Explanation: Salpingitis is the medical term for inflammation of the Fallopian tubes. The Fallopian tubes are two narrow tubes that transport the egg from the ovary to the uterus. They are also known as oviducts. Oophoritis is the medical term for inflammation of the ovary. The two female reproductive organs that create eggs are the ovaries. Both salpingitis and oophoritis can be caused by infection. Infections that cause salpingitis or oophoritis can be sexually transmitted, such as chlamydia or gonorrhea. They can also be caused by other types of infections, such as those that occur after pelvic surgery. Symptoms of salpingitis or oophoritis include pain in the lower abdomen, fever, and abnormal vaginal discharge.

Question 126:
Answer :
C. vernix
Explanation: Vernix is a thick substance that is waxy and is present between fetal skin and the amniotic sac. It is thought to protect the fetus from the amniotic fluid and from the outside world. It is also thought to help keep the fetus warm.

Question 127:
Answer:

B. Uterine atony.

Explanation: When the uterus fails to contract after childbirth, it is called uterine atony. This dangerous disorder has the potential to cause significant bleeding. Without contractions, the uterus cannot push the blood out and blood clots can form. If the bleeding is severe, it can be life-threatening. Uterine atony is the most common cause of postpartum hemorrhage (PPH), which is excessive bleeding after childbirth. PPH is defined as blood loss of more than 500 mL (about two cups) within the first 24 hours after delivery. While PPH can happen during vaginal or cesarean births, it is more common after vaginal delivery.

Question 128:
Answer:

A.Firm.

EXPLANATION: After delivery, the uterus should be firm. This is because the firmness of the uterus helps to keep the cervix closed, which in turn helps to prevent infection. Additionally, the firmness of the uterus aids in the involution process, during which the uterus shrinks back to its pre-pregnancy size. Without firmness, the process of involution would be delayed and the risk of infection would be greater.

Question 129:
Answer :

D. Postpartum hemorrhage

Explanation: PPH is a life-threatening condition that can occur after childbirth. It is the most common cause of maternal death worldwide. PPH occurs when there is heavy bleeding from the vagina after delivery. The bleeding can occur during labor or delivery, or it can occur up to 24 hours after delivery. PP certainly hemorrhage, or postpartum hemorrhage, is a gynecological emergency that requires immediate medical attention. It is the most common cause of maternal mortality (death) around the world. In the United States, PPH occurs in up to 4% of vaginal births and in up to 18% of cesarean births. However, the overall risk of PPH is lower in the US than in many other countries.

Question 130:
answer: Option

A) Neonatal abstinence syndrome

Explanation: A pregnant patient who has a history of drug abuse is likely to have a child with neonatal abstinence syndrome. This is a condition where the child has difficulty adapting to life outside the womb and experiences withdrawal symptoms. The symptoms can include tremors, irritability, poor feeding, and respiratory distress. Neonatal abstinence syndrome can be a very serious condition and can lead to death if not treated properly. Treatment typically includes providing supportive care and symptom management.

Question 131:
answer: Option

A) Maternal fever

Explanation: Fetal tachycardia is a condition in which the fetal heart rate is abnormally fast. It is mostly seen in cases where the mother has a fever. This is because the fever can cause the fetal heart rate to increase. In some cases, the fetal heart rate may also increase due to other factors, such as maternal smoking or the use of illicit drugs. Fetal tachycardia can be a sign of a serious condition, such as infection, and it is important for pregnant women to seek medical attention if they experience this symptom.

Question 132

Answer:
 A.Improve the oxygen supply to the fetus
EXPLANATION: A medical disorder called hypertension causes high blood pressure. The force of the blood against the artery walls is known as blood pressure. The higher the blood pressure, the greater the risk of heart disease, stroke, and kidney disease. A pregnant woman who is hypertensive is at risk for a number of complications, including premature birth, low birth weight, and stillbirth. In addition, hypertension can lead to placental abruption, in which the placenta separates from the uterus prematurely. Hypertension can be caused by a number of factors, including obesity, diabetes, and kidney disease. It is important to control hypertension during pregnancy to reduce the risk of complications.

Question 133:

Answer:
 A. Let-down reflex.
 Explanation: The let-down reflex is the reflex that stimulates the cells of the breast to eject the milk out. This reflex is triggered by the sound of the baby crying, the touch of the baby's lips on the nipple, or the sight of the baby. The let-down reflex is a conditioned reflex, which means that it is learned. In the early days after birth, the let-down reflex may not be strong enough to eject the milk. The mother may need to massage her breast or use a breast pump to help the reflex along.

Question 134:

 Answer: A. Microcephaly
EXPLANATION:
When a pregnant woman goes in for an ultrasound scan typically at around the start of her ninth week of gestation, doctors may find signs of a fetus that is developing abnormally. This could be due to a variety of medical conditions, some of which can be minor, some of which can cause serious problems for the mother and her baby. In this case, a deformed fetus is found on the scan, which can lead to a range of issues for the baby when it is born.

One of the most common consequences of a deformed fetus is an issue with the structure and/or function of the internal organs. This can cause issues such as cardiac defects, digestive problems, and problems with the central nervous system and the development of the brain. Such issues can cause health problems and learning and behavioral difficulties that can last into adulthood. Other issues that may result from this type of abnormality include cleft lip and/or palate, clubfoot, and other limb deformities. Microcephaly is not a birth defect arising from a deformed fetus. **Question 135:**

Answer:

B.Fetal head compression

EXPLANATION: One of the risk factors for the fetus during parturition is fetal head compression. This can occur when the fetus is pushed down into the pelvis during labor and the head is compressed. This can result in the baby's head being misshapen or deformed. During parturition, it is important to monitor the fetus for any signs of distress. If the fetus is showing signs of distress, such as a decrease in heart rate, it may be necessary to perform a C-section to deliver the baby. Fetal head compression is a risk factor for the fetus during parturition, but it can be managed with close monitoring and interventions if necessary.

Question 136

Answer:

B. Hyperemesis gravidarum.

EXPLANATION: A disorder known as hyperemesis gravidarum (HG) during pregnancy is characterized by intense nausea and vomiting. HG can lead to dehydration and weight loss and can be very debilitating. Women with HG frequently have to miss work and might not be able to look after their other children. HG can also cause anxiety and depression. Morning sickness is a normal part of pregnancy, but for women with HG, it can be much more severe. There is no one cause of HG, but it is thought to be related to the high levels of hormones in pregnancy. HG is more common in first-time pregnancies and in multiple pregnancies. It is also more common in women who have a history of motion sickness or nausea and vomiting. Treatment for HG typically involves relieving symptoms and preventing dehydration. Anti-nausea medications can be helpful, but some women may need IV fluids to prevent dehydration. HG usually goes away after the first trimester, but some women may experience symptoms throughout their pregnancy.

Question 137:

Answer:

B. 200ml

Explanation: A unit of pRBCs contains around 200ml of blood. This is a relatively small amount, which makes it easier to transfuse pRBCs into a person than to transfuse whole blood. pRBCs are often transfused when a person has lost a lot of blood, such as during surgery. They are also sometimes given to people who have anemia, a condition in which the person does not have enough RBCs. Giving pRBCs to people with anemia can help to improve their symptoms.

Question 138
Answer:

D. Bacteria.

Explanation An infection of the urinary system, which includes the kidneys, ureters, bladder, and urethra, is known as a urinary tract infection (UTI). UTIs are usually caused by bacteria. Burning or pain when peeing is the most typical sign of a UTI. Other symptoms may include urgency to urinate, cloudy or bloody urine, or strong-smelling urine. If the infection spreads to the kidneys, it can cause fever, back pain, and vomiting. UTIs are treated with antibiotics. If the infection is severe, hospitalization may be necessary. Bacteria are the most common cause of UTIs. Escherichia coli is the most prevalent form of bacteria that causes UTIs (E. coli). Other types of bacteria that can cause UTIs include Staphylococcus, Streptococcus, and Klebsiella.

Question 139:

Answer:
C.   Wharton's Jelly envelops the umbilical cord, provides cushioning effect, and protects the umbilical cord .

EXPLANATION: Wharton's jelly cushions and protects the blood vessels within the umbilical cord. The umbilical cord is a conducting passage between the fetus and the placenta and contains the blood vessels that carry oxygen and nutrients to the fetus. The umbilical cord is surrounded by a layer of connective tissue called Wharton's jelly. This jelly cushions and protects the blood vessels, and helps to prevent them from becoming twisted or kinked.

Question 140:

Answer:
D. Placenta percreta

EXPLANATION: Placenta percreta is considered a perforation of the uterus caused by the placenta. This occurs when the placenta grows into the uterine wall, penetrating the muscle and possibly other organs. This can happen during pregnancy or delivery. Placenta percreta is a serious complication that can lead to maternal hemorrhage, uterine rupture, and even death. Treatment typically involves delivering the baby as soon as possible and then surgically removing the placenta.

Question 141:

Answer:
C.Uterine rupture.

EXPLANATION: If a pregnant woman presents with severe abdominal pain and tachycardia, it is most likely a case of uterine rupture. This is a serious complication that can occur during pregnancy, labor, or delivery. If the uterine ruptures, the baby can be expelled from the womb and into the abdomen. This can lead to serious maternal and fetal complications, including death. The best way to prevent uterine rupture is to get regular prenatal care and to be aware of the signs and symptoms.

Question 142

.

Answer:
D.   Miscarriage and early delivery.

Explanation: Listeriosis is a foodborne illness that can be passed from mother to fetus during pregnancy. The bacteria that cause listeriosis, Listeria monocytogenes, are found in contaminated food, including raw milk and soft cheeses. Pregnant women are 20 times more likely than the general population to contract listeriosis, and the infection can lead to miscarriage, stillbirth, or premature delivery. Listeriosis is thought to cause miscarriage by infecting the placenta, causing inflammation, and preventing the transfer of oxygen and nutrients to the fetus. The infection can also lead to premature labor and delivery, as the body attempts to expel the contaminated fetus. In severe cases, listeriosis can cause fetal death. Listeriosis is a serious infection, and pregnant women should take care to avoid foods that may be contaminated with Listeria monocytogenes. Pregnant women should also avoid unpasteurized milk and cheeses, as well as deli meats and hot dogs unless they are heated to steaming hot before consumption.

Question 143:

Answer:
B. Weight of the fetus.

Explanation: A 39 year old female patient is pregnant and in her late stage of pregnancy. oligohydramnios is a complication that can occur during pregnancy, and it can lead to a number of complications for the mother and baby. The weight of the fetus is not a complication of oligohydramnios. Some of the potential complications of oligohydramnios include decreased fetal movement, small for gestational-age babies, preterm labor, and placental abruption. oligohydramnios can also cause the baby to be in a breech position. If a woman has oligohydramnios, her doctor will likely monitor her closely and may recommend a course of treatment. Treatment options for oligohydramnios include increased hydration, bed rest, and in some cases, induction of labor.

Question 144:

Answer:
B. Doppler ultrasound of the lower extremities.

Explanation: Deep vein thrombosis (DVT) is a condition that can occur after childbirth. A blood clot known as a DVT develops in a vein, typically in the leg.. DVT is a serious condition because the clot can break free and travel to the lungs, causing a blockage (pulmonary embolism). There are several tests that can be used to diagnose DVT, but the most common and most reliable test is Doppler ultrasound. This test uses sound waves to create a picture of the blood flow in the veins. The doctor will look for areas of the veins that are not flowing well, which can indicate a clot. Doppler ultrasound is considered the gold standard for diagnosing DVT, and it is the most accurate test available. It is also the best test for ruling out DVT, meaning that if the test is negative, it is very unlikely that the person has DVT.

Question 145:
Answer:
D.   5 or fewer contractions in 10 minutes, lasting about 60 seconds.

EXPLANATION: When a woman is in her 39th week of pregnancy, she is considered to be in the active phase of labor. This is the phase when the contractions become more frequent, intense, and regular. The pattern of contractions during this phase is usually 5 or fewer contractions in 10 minutes, lasting about 60 seconds. The contractions during the active phase of labor help to open the cervix and push the baby down into the birth canal. This is the most important phase of labor, and it is when the majority of the progress is made. The active phase usually lasts for about 3-4 hours, but it can vary from woman to woman.

Question 146

Answer:

B. Tonic neck reflex.

Explanation: When a newborn is lying on their back and their head turns to one side, this is known as the tonic neck reflex. This reflex is also sometimes called the fencing reflex or the Moro reflex. It is a primitive reflex that is present at birth and typically disappears by 4-6 months of age. This reflex is thought to be a vestigial remnant of a time when our ancestors were quadrupedal. When an animal is lying on its side, the position of the limbs helps to prevent the animal from rolling over onto its back. The tonic neck reflex may help newborns maintain this position so that they do not roll over and become stuck on their backs, which would make it difficult to breathe.

Question 147:

Answer :

B. financial status of the mother

Explanation When a mother gives birth, she and her infant go through a period of adjustment as they get to know each other and form a bond. This bonding process is important for the infant's development and well-being, and it begins with a behavior called attachment. Attachment is the special relationship that develops between an infant and their primary caregiver, usually the mother. It is characterized by the infant seeking proximity to the mother and is thought to be important for the infant's survival. The attachment behavior period is the time from birth until around six months of age when the infant is most active in seeking proximity to the mother. There are several factors that contribute to the development of attachment, including the mother's responsiveness to the infant's needs, the physical closeness between the two, and the infant's own temperament. The mother's financial status does not play a role in attachment behavior. There are different types of attachment, but all involve the infant using the mother (or primary caregiver) as a "secure base" from which to explore the world.

Question 148

Answer :

D. Afterpains

Explanation: The term given to define sporadic uterine contractions is 'afterpains'. Afterpains are usually harmless and do not require any medical treatment, though they may be accompanied by cramping and discomfort. Although they can arise in the days or weeks following childbirth, they often happen right after delivery. Many women report that afterpains feel like strong menstrual cramps. Afterpains are caused by the uterus shrinking back to its pre-pregnancy size. This process is helped by the hormone oxytocin, which is released during breastfeeding. As the uterus returns to its normal size, it puts pressure on the surrounding organs, which can cause cramping. Afterpains are more likely to occur after a woman delivers a baby vaginally, as opposed to via c-section. They are also more likely to occur if the woman is breastfeeding. There are a few things that women can do to help relieve afterpains. Taking a warm bath or using a heating pad on the abdomen can help to ease cramping.

Question 149:

Answer:
A. Sexually transmitted disease.
Explanation: Bacterial vaginosis (BV) is a condition that can occur in women of any age. It is caused by an imbalance of the bacteria that are normally present in the vagina. BV is not a sexually transmitted disease (STD), but it is associated with sexual activity. Women who have never had sexual intercourse can also get BV. The most typical vaginal infection in women who are fertile is BV. It is also the most common reason for women to have an abnormal vaginal discharge. BV is usually not a serious condition, but it can cause discomfort and sometimes lead to other problems. The most common symptom of BV is a vaginal discharge that has a fishy smell. The discharge may be white or gray and may be thin or watery.

Question 150:

Answer:
D. Increase bed rest and low physical activity.
Explanation: Placenta previa is a condition where the placenta partially or totally covers the cervical opening. When it occurs without bleeding, it is considered a low-risk condition. However, bed rest and low physical activity are still recommended treatments. The purpose of bed rest is to decrease the amount of blood flow to the uterus. This is important because placenta previa can cause bleeding. Low physical activity helps to decrease the amount of blood flow to the uterus as well. If bleeding does occur, it is important to seek medical help.

Question 151:

Answer:
A.Day three

EXPLANATION: It is common for a woman's bowel sounds to be more audible on day three postpartum. This is due to the increased gas and feces present in the intestines as the body continues to expel waste from the delivery. The peristalsis, or muscular contractions, of the intestines, are also more pronounced as the intestines return to their normal state. Amelia may notice that her bowel movements are not as regular as they were pre-pregnancy. This is because the pregnancy hormones that slow down the digestive system are still present. It is important for Amelia to take laxatives or stool softeners if she is having difficulty passing stool. She should also drink plenty of fluids and eat high-fiber foods to help keep her bowel movements regular.

Question 152
answer: Option
C)both a and b
Explanation: A smooth, regular pattern that resembles a wave on a fetal heart monitor is indicative of a healthy pregnancy. In this case, the mother is Rh negative and the child is Rh positive. This can pose a problem because if the mother's body produces antibodies against the Rh factor, it can cross the placenta and attack the baby's red blood cells. This can cause anemia, which can be serious or even fatal. However, if the mother has had a previous child who was Rh positive, she is likely to have already developed immunity to the Rh factor and will not produce antibodies. In this case, both the mother and the child are healthy and the pregnancy is progressing normally.

Question 153:
Answer:
C. Raw fruits.
Explanation: When it comes to pregnancy, there are a lot of things that women are told to avoid. Everything from certain foods to certain activities can be off-limits when you're expecting. But when it comes to raw fruits, there's no need to avoid them. In fact, raw fruits can actually be very good for you during pregnancy. Raw fruits are a great source of vitamins and minerals. They include a lot of fiber, which might keep you regular. They're a healthy alternative to snacks like cookies or chips.

Question 154:

Answer:
D. Abruptio placenta
EXPLANATION: Placental abruption is a complication of pregnancy in which the placenta partially or completely separates from the wall of the uterus before delivery. It occurs in about 1 in 150 pregnancies. Symptoms of placental abruption can include bleeding from the vagina, abdominal pain, back pain, and uterine tenderness. If the abruption is severe, it can lead to shock and even death. While the exact cause of placental abruption is unknown, it is thought to be caused by a combination of factors, including smoking, hypertension, trauma, and placental abnormalities.

Question 155:

answer) Option
A) the baby's head is known to be engaged or aligned with the ischial spine
Explanation:

When a woman is in labor, her body is going through intense changes as her baby moves down the birth canal. The baby's head is known to be engaged or aligned with the ischial spine, which is the lower part of the pelvis near the tailbone, by the time she is at zero station. This is an important indicator of how far along labor is progressing and how close the baby is to being born. Engagement is when the widest diameter of the fetal head has passed below the pubic arch and is lying in the pelvic cavity. This typically happens sometime during the last few weeks of pregnancy but can occur earlier or later depending on the individual. Once engaged, the baby's head becomes fixed in one position and can no longer move up or down in the birth canal. Zero station is the point at which the baby's head is at the level of the ischial spines, or in other words, the baby's head is as low as it can go in the pelvis.

Question 156
answer: Option
D)Both a and c
Explanation: Ultrasound scanning is most commonly performed transabdominal and transurethral during the second trimester of pregnancy, but can be done earlier in the pregnancy if there are concerns about the baby's development. The ultrasound allows the doctor to see how the baby is growing and to check for any problems. The ultrasound can also be used to determine the baby's gender if the parents want to know. Ultrasound scanning is considered safe for both the mother and the baby.

Question 157

answer) Option
    A.   Cervix is closed and is firm

Explanation: Cervical insufficiency, also known as cervical incompetence, is a condition that can lead to late-term pregnancy loss. The uterus's lower, more narrow end, which opens into the vagina, is known as the cervix. The cervix normally is firm and has a closed opening. In cervical insufficiency, the cervix begins to open too early during the pregnancy, often before the baby is ready to be born. This condition can occur when the cervix is weakened or stretched and can no longer support the weight of the growing baby. Cervical insufficiency often is caused by a problem with the structure or function of the cervix. The cervix may be weak or shortened. Damage to the cervix also may occur from surgery, such as a cone biopsy or loop electrosurgical excision procedure (LEEP). Cervical insufficiency usually is diagnosed after a woman has had two or more late-term pregnancy losses.

Question 158:

Answer:
A. Artifact.
Explanation: Artifact is the right term for the extra noise that is created when the mother and baby are moving together. This is because the noise is created by the movement of the two bodies and is not an inherent property of either the mother or the baby.

Question 159:

Answer:

A.Aneuploidy.

Explanation: Aneuploidy refers to a situation in which there is an abnormal number of chromosomes. This can happen for a variety of reasons, but the end result is that the individual will have genetic defects. The most common form of aneuploidy is Down syndrome, which occurs when there is an extra copy of chromosome 21. This extra chromosome leads to a variety of physical and mental defects. Other forms of aneuploidy can also cause serious defects and even death.

Question 160:

Answer:
C. Infections of the middle ear

EXPLANATION. A cleft palate is an opening in the roof of the mouth that can occur when the tissues that make up the roof of the mouth do not fuse together properly during development. This opening can allow food and liquids to enter the nose, which can lead to middle-ear infections. The risk of middle-ear infections is higher in children and newborns with cleft palates because they are more likely to have an opening between the nose and the throat, which allows bacteria to enter the middle ear.

Question 161:
Answer:
C. No earlier pregnancy or uterine surgeries.
.

Explanation: Placenta previa is a condition in which the placenta partially or completely covers the cervix. Women who have had no previous pregnancies or uterine surgeries are not at risk for placenta previa. The most common symptom of placenta previa is bleeding during the second or third trimester of pregnancy. This bleeding can be heavy and may require hospitalization. Placenta previa can also cause premature labor and delivery. Placenta previa is diagnosed through ultrasound. Treatment depends on the severity of the condition and may include bed rest, blood transfusions, and steroids to mature the baby's lungs. A cesarean delivery could be required in specific circumstances.

Question 162
Answer:
C.Gonorrhea

EXPLANATION: There are a variety of factors that can contribute to a baby being born with low birth weight (under 5.5 pounds). Some of these factors include:
-Maternal age: Women who are younger than 20 or older than 35 are more likely to have a baby with low birth weight.
-Smoking: Women who smoke during pregnancy are more likely to have a baby with low birth weight.
-Alcohol use: Women who drink alcohol during pregnancy are more likely to have a baby with low birth weight.
-Illegal drug use: Women who use illegal drugs during pregnancy are more likely to have a baby with low birth weight.
-Medical conditions: Women with certain medical conditions, such as diabetes or high blood pressure, are more likely to have a baby with low birth weight.
-Multiple births: Women who have twins or triplets are more likely to have a baby with low birth weight.

-Premature birth: Women who give birth before 37 weeks of pregnancy are more likely to have a baby with low birth

Question 163:

Answer:
A. Kidney failure.
Explanation: The postpartum period is a time of great physical and emotional transition for a woman. It is also a time when her body is changing and healing from the arduous process of childbirth. There are many risks associated with the postpartum period, but kidney failure is not one of them. The most common risks during this time include: 1. Haemorrhage: Excessive bleeding (hemorrhage) post-delivery is one of the most serious complications facing women during the postpartum period. It is crucial that all women are monitored closely for excessive bleeding, as it can lead to death if left untreated. 2. Infection: Childbirth can be a dirty business, and infection is one of the most common risks during the postpartum.

Question 164:
Answer: Fidelity.
Explanation
The regulations under the Health Insurance Portability and Accountability Act (HIPAA) require medical professionals to maintain the confidentiality of patients' protected health information (PHI). This is commonly referred to as the "fidelity" principle. The HIPAA Privacy Rule establishes national standards to protect individuals' PHI. The Rule requires covered entities to take reasonable steps to safeguard PHI from unauthorized uses or disclosures. Covered entities include health plans, healthcare clearinghouses, and healthcare providers that conduct certain transactions electronically. Medical professionals are bound by the HIPAA Security Rule to implement security measures to protect PHI. The Security Rule requires covered entities to put in place physical, administrative, and technical safeguards to protect the confidentiality, integrity, and availability of PHI. Physical safeguards are measures to protect electronic PHI from unauthorized physical access. Administrative safeguards are measures to protect against unauthorized uses and disclosures of PHI. Technical safeguards are measures to protect electronic PHI from unauthorized access and to ensure its integrity.

Question 165:

Answer:
E. Glucose test.
Explanation ultrasound test is usually conducted with other tests to diagnose polyhydramnios. A glucose test is one of the tests used to diagnose polyhydramnios. A condition called polyhydramnios occurs when there is too much amniotic fluid in the womb. This can happen for a number of reasons, including diabetes in the mother, twins or triplets, or genetic abnormalities in the baby. The extra fluid can cause the womb to expand more than normal, and the baby may have trouble moving around. They may also be at risk of compression of the umbilical cord, which can reduce the blood flow and oxygen supply to the baby.

Question 166
Answer:

C. Cool air vents.

Explanation: Convection is the process by which heat is transferred from the body to the surrounding air. The rate of convection is determined by the difference in temperature between the body and the surrounding air, as well as the wind speed. When the body is in a cold environment, the rate of convection is increased and the body loses heat more quickly. The newborn infant is particularly vulnerable to convective heat loss because their skin is thin and they have a large body surface area relative to their size. The main way that a newborn infant can lose body heat through convection is by exposure to cool air vents. When the infant is placed in a crib near a vent, the cool air blowing from the vent will cause the infant's body temperature to drop.

Question 167:

Answer:

B.Striae

EXPLANATION: Stretch marks, also called striae, are markings that commonly show up on the skin during periods of rapid growth or weight gain. Stretch marks can occur on anyone, but they are most common in women during pregnancy or puberty. When the skin stretches too quickly, the collagen and elastin fibers that make up the skin's supportive structure can break down, resulting in stretch marks. There are several ways to treat stretch marks, but unfortunately, there is no way to completely remove them. However, there are treatments that can help to make them less visible. Common treatments include topical creams and laser therapy.

Question 168:

Answer :

B. Overt

Explanation : Cord prolapse is the most common type of birth injury. It occurs when the umbilical cord is compressed, preventing blood and oxygen from reaching the baby. This can lead to serious health problems for the baby, including brain damage and even death. There are two types of cord prolapse: overt and covert. Overt cord prolapse is when the cord is visibly prolapsed, typically before the baby has crowned. Covert cord prolapse is when the cord is compressed but not visible. It is often only discovered after the baby has been born. Overt cord prolapse is more common than covert cord prolapse and is more likely to cause serious health problems for the baby.

Question 169:

Answer:

C. Vaginal Birth After Cesarean.

Explanation: A cesarean delivery, also known as a C-section, is a surgical procedure in which the baby is born through an incision in the mother's abdomen. A vaginal birth after a cesarean (VBAC) is a vaginal delivery that occurs after a woman has previously had a cesarean delivery. The American College of Obstetricians and Gynecologists (ACOG) released new guidelines in 2010 stating that a trial of labor after cesarean delivery (TOLAC) is a safe and appropriate option for most women who have had a previous cesarean delivery. In general, a woman who has had a cesarean delivery can attempt a vaginal birth as long as the following criteria are met: The previous cesarean delivery was performed through a low transverse incision. The woman is currently pregnant with a singleton fetus in a vertex (head-first) position. The woman has no contraindications to labor, such as placenta previa.

Question 170:

Answer:
A.Gastrulation.
Explanation: Gastrulation is one of the earlier stages of embryo development for most animals. During this, a single-layered hollow sphere of cells is formed called blastula. This is later reorganized into a multilayered structure called the gastrula. Gastrulation occurs after cleavage and formation of the blastula. Gastrulation is the biological process that creates the mesoderm. This early phase in embryonic development occurs when a single blastula becomes a trilaminar. The ectoderm, mesoderm, and endoderm are created during gastrulation. Gastrulation is a crucial stage in embryogenesis, during which the three germ layers of the embryo are formed. It is a complex process, involving coordinated cell movements that result in the formation of the ectoderm, mesoderm, and endoderm.

Question 171:

Answer:
A.   Erythromycin
EXPLANATION: Neisseria gonorrhea is a sexually transmitted infection (STI) caused by the bacteria Neisseria gonorrhoeae. This bacteria can infect the genitals, rectum, and throat. Symptoms in newborns can include red and swollen eyes, thick purulent discharge from the eyes, and eye irritation. An antibiotic called erythromycin is used to treat bacterial infections.. It works by stopping the growth of bacteria. Erythromycin is used to treat infections of the skin, ears, respiratory tract, and eyes. Additionally, it's employed to avoid bacterial endocarditis. The drug erythromycin belongs to the group of drugs known as macrolide antibiotics.

Question 172:

Answer:
A.   Preterm birth and low birth weight.
EXPLANATION: During pregnancy, the demand for iron increases as the baby grows. The placenta also takes iron from the mother to support the baby's development. If a pregnant woman doesn't have enough iron in her diet, she can develop iron deficiency anemia. This can lead to serious health problems for both the mother and the baby. Iron deficiency anemia during pregnancy is associated with an increased risk of preterm birth and low birth weight. Preterm birth is when a baby is born before 37 weeks of gestation. Low birth weight is when a baby is born weighing less than 5.5 pounds (2.5 kg). Babies born prematurely are at higher risk for a number of health problems, including respiratory distress, feeding difficulties, and jaundice. They are also more likely to experience developmental delays.

Question 173:

Answer:
F.   3 months

EXPLANATION: Doppler ultrasound is a type of ultrasound that uses sound waves to assess the blood flow in the vessels. It can be used to assess the fetal heart rate and development of organs. Doppler ultrasound is indicated after 3 months of pregnancy. During a Doppler ultrasound, the transducer emits sound waves that bounce off of moving objects, such as red blood cells. The Doppler effect is the difference in the frequency of the sound waves that are received by the transducer when the object is moving towards the transducer, and when the object is moving away from the transducer. This difference in frequency is used to calculate the velocity of the object. Doppler ultrasound can be used to assess the fetal heart rate and development of organs.

Question 174:

Answer:
D.All of the above
EXPLANATION: Fetal tachycardia is defined as a heart rate greater than 180 beats per minute and is considered to be a sign of potential fetal distress. There are many factors that can lead to fetal tachycardia, including maternal fever, maternal hyperthyroidism, infection, dehydration, or anemia. Additionally, maternal smoking, drug use, or exposure to environmental toxins can also lead to fetal tachycardia. Placental insufficiency, twin-to-twin transfusion syndrome, or other congenital heart defects can also cause fetal tachycardia.

Question 175:

Answer:
A.8 to 18.
Explanation:
The amount of amniotic fluid present in a pregnant woman's uterus varies throughout pregnancy. In the early stages of pregnancy, there is typically a small amount of amniotic fluid present. As the pregnancy progresses, the amount of amniotic fluid gradually increases. By the end of the pregnancy, the amount of amniotic fluid typically ranges from 8 to 18. The amount of amniotic fluid can be affected by various factors. For example, if a pregnant woman has a condition called oligohydramnios, it means that she has a low amount of amniotic fluid. This can be caused by factors such as premature rupture of membranes (PROM) or leaky valves in the pregnant woman's veins.

Question 176:

Answer :
C. to develop NCLEX RN and PN licensing exam
Explanation: National Council of State Boards of Nursing (NCSBN) is set up to develop NCLEX RN and PN licensing exams, as well as to provide research-based recommendations for nursing education and practice. The organization is made up of representatives from all 50 U.S. states. NCSBN develops both the NCLEX-RN and NCLEX-PN exams, which are used by all U.S. states and jurisdictions to license registered nurses and practical/vocational nurses, respectively. In addition to developing and administering these exams, NCSBN provides recommendations on minimum educational requirements for licensure, as well as guidance on the management of licensure records.

Question 177:

 answer: Option
 D.both b and c

 Explanation: As a nurse, you play a vital role in EFM by educating patients on the need for this treatment and recording the results of EFM. EFM is a process of monitoring a fetus's heart rate and contractions during labor. This information is then used to make decisions about the care of the mother and baby. The benefits of EFM include:

1. Better outcomes for mothers and babies.
2. Early identification of problems with the baby's heart rate or contractions.
3. Reduced risk of oxygen deprivation for the baby.
4. shorter labor and delivery times.
5. Reduced risk of cesarean delivery.

In addition, you will be responsible for recording the results of EFM and providing this information to the physician.

Question 178:

Answer:

A. preterm birth
   EXPLANATION: A woman's risk for preterm birth increases if she has a urinary tract infection. Burning during urination and cloudy or smelly urine are both symptoms of a UTI. The infection can cause the woman's cervix to become inflamed, which can lead to preterm labor. A UTI is a serious infection and must be treated quickly to reduce the risk of preterm birth.

Question 179

Answer:
C. 3 - 4 days.
 Explanation: It's common for a mother's milk to "come in" 3 to 4 days after her baby is born. However, occasionally it could take a bit longer. This is because a mother's body is making milk for her baby and it can take a few days for her body to get the rhythm of milk production going. During this time, it's important to continue to breastfeed or pump your breasts regularly (8 to 12 times a day), even if you don't see much milk coming out at first. This will help signal your body to make more milk.

Question 180

Answer: A . Diamond and open shaped
 Explanation: The fontanelles are two soft spots on a newborn's head. There are two fontanelles: - Anterior (front): This fontanelle is often diamond-shaped and is located at the top front of the head - Posterior (back): This fontanelle is larger, more triangular, and located at the back of the head. Both fontanelles allow the rapid growth of the brain during infancy and childhood and provide flexibility to the skull. The posterior fontanelle usually closes between two and eight weeks after birth, while the anterior fontanelle usually closes between six and eighteen months after birth.

Question 181:

Answer:

A. Pelvic outlet.

Explanation: The pelvic outlet is an important part of the maternal pelvis. It is the outlet for the fetus during childbirth. The pelvic outlet is located between the pubic symphysis and the coccyx. It is important for the pelvic outlet to be large enough for the fetus to pass through during childbirth.

Question 182:

Answer:

A. 10.

Explanation: When a baby is born, they take their first breath and begin to breathe on their own. Before this happens, the baby's oxygen saturation levels start to drop. This happens because the baby's oxygen levels are lower than the mother's levels. The baby's oxygen levels start to decrease as they move through the birth canal and their head starts to emerge. The baby's oxygen levels continue to decrease until they take their first breath and start to breathe on their own. The percentage of fetal oxygen saturation that drops during labor is around 10%.

Question 183:
Answer:

D. Empty urinary bladder.

EXPLANATION: Involution is the process by which the uterus returns to its non-pregnant state. It is known to be slowed by a number of factors, including: - Obesity - Poor nutrition - Stress - Smoking However, one factor that is known to speed up involution is an empty urinary bladder. This is because the act of urinating helps to expel any residual blood and tissue from the uterus, helping it to return to its normal size and shape more quickly.

Question 184:

Answer:

B. Neonatal lupus.

Explanation: When a baby is born, its mother's condition of lupus may lead to the baby being born prematurely. If the baby is born prematurely, it may suffer from neonatal lupus. Neonatal lupus is a rare condition that can occur when the mother has lupus. The condition can cause a rash on the baby's face, body, and scalp. It can also cause the baby to have a low birth weight. In some cases, neonatal lupus can cause heart problems in the baby. treatment for neonatal lupus depends on the severity of the condition. The most common treatment is to keep the baby away from sunlight. If the condition is more severe, the baby may need to be treated with steroids.

Question 185:
answer: Option

B) It is borderline high and requires evaluation

Explanation: If the normal resting tone of the uterus is 20 mm hg, the conclusion is that it is borderline high and requires evaluation. The uterus is a muscle that contracts and relaxes to help deliver babies during childbirth. The resting tone of the uterus is the tone of the muscle when it is not contracting. A normal resting tone is between 10 and 20 mm hg. A tone that is borderline high is between 20 and 25 mm hg. A tone that is high is over 25 mm hg. A high tone can be a sign of a problem with the uterus, such as a fibroid tumor. If the tone is high, it is important to see a doctor for an evaluation.

Question 186

Answer:
B. 3.
Explanation: There are three levels of cues when an infant is ready to nurse: visual, auditory, and olfactory. Visual cues include the infant's rooting reflex, where the infant turns its head towards a stimulus, and the sucking reflex, where the infant rhythmically sucks on anything that enters its mouth. Auditory cues include the sound of the mother's heartbeat and the sound of her voice. Olfactory cues include the smell of the mother's milk and the smell of her skin.

Question 187:

Answer:
A. Fifth degree.
Explanation: An episiotomy is a surgical incision made in the perineum, the area between the vagina and anus, in order to widen the vaginal opening. This is typically done during childbirth in order to prevent tissue tearing. There are four degrees of episiotomy, ranging from a first degree, which is a small incision made in the perineum, to a fourth degree, which is a large incision that extends into the anal canal. A fifth-degree episiotomy is even more severe and involves an incision that extends through the anal sphincter. This degree of episiotomy is very rare and is only done in exceptional circumstances.

Question 188:

Answer: Calf pain when the foot is dorsiflexed
EXPLANATION: Homan's sign is a clinical sign that is elicited during a physical examination. It is used to help diagnose deep vein thrombosis (DVT), which is a blood clot that forms in the deep veins of the body, usually in the legs. The sign is named after Dr. Frederick W. Homan, who described it in a paper published in 1928. To elicit Homan's sign, the examiner stands behind the patient and grasps the patient's calf. The patient's leg is then flexed at the knee and extended at the ankle so that the foot is dorsiflexed. The examiner then applies gentle but firm pressure on the calf. If the patient has DVT, this maneuver will cause pain in the calf.

Question 189:
Answer:
D.   Organomegaly

EXPLANATION: While evaluating the overall health of a fetus, biophysical variables such as heart rate, breathing, and muscle tone will be assessed. These variables can provide insight into how the fetus is developing and help to identify any potential problems. However, there are some variables that are not used when assessing the health of a fetus. One of these is organomegaly, which refers to the enlargement of one or more organs. This can be a normal finding in some pregnancies, but it can also indicate a serious underlying condition. Therefore, it is not used as a routine part of fetal health assessment.

Question 190:

Answer:

A.Category 3

EXPLANATION: Category 3 refers to fetal assessment where there are some reassuring features and some features of concern. In this case, the baseline heart rate is changing and there are recurrent decreases in the fetal heart rate following a sinusoidal path. These features may be of concern, but there are also some reassuring features present. For example, the fact that the heart rate is changing suggests that the fetus is responding to its environment. The fact that the heart rate is following a sinusoidal path suggests that the fetus is healthy and that the changes in heart rate are not due to an underlying problem.

Question 191:

Answer:

A.Bone marrow.

Explanation: When a woman gives birth, her body expels the placenta and any leftover tissue and blood from the uterus in a process called Lochia. This discharge can last anywhere from a few days to six weeks postpartum. The Lochia will gradually change color, going from dark red to pink and then becoming white or pale yellow. Along with this change in color, the Lochia will also decrease in amount over time. The three stages of Lochia are: 1. Lochia rubra: This is the stage immediately after birth, when the discharge is heavy and bright red in color. It typically lasts for 3-5 days. 2. Lochia serosa: This stage occurs after Lochia rubra and is characterized by a lighter discharge that is pink or light brown in color. It usually lasts for 2-3 weeks. 3. Lochia alba: This is the final stage of Lochia, when the discharge is white or pale yellow and is much lighter in volume. It can last up to six weeks postpartum.

Question 192:

Answer:

A. Tachycardia.

EXPLANATION: Tachycardia is defined as a heart rate that is greater than the normal range for a particular age group. In fetuses, the normal heart rate ranges from 110-160 beats per minute. If a Doppler ultrasound reveals a heart rate above 160 beats per minute, this is considered to be tachycardia. There are several potential causes of fetal tachycardia. One possibility is that the fetus is experiencing stress or anxiety. This can cause the heart to beat faster in an attempt to pump more oxygenated blood to the body. Another possibility is that the fetus has an infection or another medical condition that is causing the heart rate to increase.

Question 193:

Answer:
B. Maternal blood rebuilding

Explanation: The postpartum period is a time when the mother's body is working to recover from the physical demands of pregnancy and childbirth. One of the ways the body does this is by rebuilding the maternal blood supply. This process requires nutrients that are found in prenatal vitamins, which is why it is important for mothers to continue taking them during the postpartum period. Prenatal vitamins contain nutrients like iron, folic acid, and vitamin B12, which are all important for the formation of new blood cells. Iron is particularly important because it is involved in the production of hemoglobin, a protein that carries oxygen in the blood. Folic acid helps to prevent birth defects of the brain and spine, and vitamin B12 is necessary for the proper function of red blood cells. By continuing to take prenatal vitamins during the postpartum period, mothers are giving their bodies the resources it needs to rebuild the blood supply and recover from childbirth.

Question 194

answer: Option
A)It may cause maternal dysphoria

Explanation: When a mother is pregnant, she can sometimes experience a feeling of sadness or depression. The hormonal changes that take place during pregnancy are to blame for this. Nubain can help to alleviate this by decreasing the levels of certain hormones in the body. However, it can also cause maternal dysphoria. This is a condition where the mother feels excessively anxious, irritable, or even depressed. This can be detrimental to both the mother and the child. Therefore, Nubain was discontinued in order to prevent this from happening.

Question 195:

Answer: Pitocin should be started at a higher dose for the patient

Explanation:

Abruptio placentae is a serious complication of pregnancy in which the placenta, the organ that provides nutrients and oxygen to the fetus, partially or completely separates from the uterine wall before delivery. This can cause fetal distress and even death. Treatment typically includes hospitalization, bed rest, and close monitoring of the mother and baby. In some cases, Pitocin, a medication that can help to stimulate uterine contractions, may be used to deliver the baby. Pitocin should not be started at a higher dose for a patient with abruptio placentae. This could cause the uterus to contract too forcefully, which could lead to further separation of the placenta and potentially cause fetal distress or death. Pitocin should be started at the lowest possible dose and titrated up as needed. Other interventions that may be used in a patient with abruptio placentae include IV fluids, blood transfusions, and oxygen therapy.

Question 196:

answer) Option
D)All of the above

Explanation) Abruptio placenta is a medical emergency in which the placenta partially or completely separates from the uterus before birth. This can cause serious problems for the mother and baby, including heavy bleeding, miscarriage, and preterm labor. If the placenta completely separates from the uterus, it is called a placental abruption. If only a part of the placenta separates, it is called a partial abruption. Placental abruption is a relatively rare condition, occurring in only about 1% of all pregnancies. However, it is one of the leading causes of maternal and fetal death. There are several risk factors for placental abruption, including smoking, substance abuse, hypertension, and trauma. Treatment usually involves hospitalization and close monitoring of the mother and baby. The placenta may occasionally need to be removed surgically.

Question 197:

Answer:
B. 1 to 2 weeks
   EXPLANATION:
   The first step in the identification of PKU babies is the screening within the first 24 hours of life. This screening is performed by measuring the level of phenylalanine in the blood. If the level of phenylalanine is high, the baby is referred for further testing. The second step is the rescreening at 1 to 2 weeks of age. This rescreening is performed by measuring the level of phenylalanine in the blood and urine. If the level of phenylalanine in the blood is high and the level of phenylalanine in the urine is low, the baby is diagnosed with PKU.

Question 198:

Answer:
D.All of the above
EXPLANATION: Sickle cell disease is a condition in which the shape of red blood cells is affected. The red blood cells are crescent or sickle-shaped. This can happen when there is not enough oxygen in the blood. The sickle-shaped cells can get stuck in small blood vessels and block them. This can cause pain, swelling, and shortness of breath.
The disease is inherited, which means it is passed down from parents to children. It is more common in people of African descent, but it can also occur in people of other ethnicities.
Prenatal screening can be used to determine if a person has the sickle cell trait. This is a test that is done during pregnancy. If the test is positive, it means the person has the trait but does not have the disease.

Question 199:

Answer:
C. It is due to the triggering of the autonomic nervous system

EXPLANATION: During pregnancy, it is important for the mother to monitor the health of her unborn child. One way to do this is by assessing for fetal kicks. Fetal kicks are often an indication of the baby's well-being and can be used to monitor the baby's health. Fetal kicks are usually caused by the baby's movement in the womb. This movement can trigger the autonomic nervous system, which is responsible for the fight-or-flight response. The autonomic nervous system is what allows the body to automatically respond to stressful situations. When the autonomic nervous system is triggered, it can cause the mother to feel a sudden jolt or movement from the baby. This sensation is often described as feeling like a flutter, thump, or flicker. The sensation can vary in intensity, depending on the amount of movement the baby is making. Fetal kicks are often most noticeable when the mother is resting or lying down.

Question 200

Answer:

A. Slow dilation of cervix

EXPLANATION: When a woman is in labor, her uterus contracts to help push the baby out. These contractions usually start weak and then get stronger and closer together as labor progresses. However, in some cases, labor can be prolonged or "stalled‿ due to weak contractions. This is known as protracted or prolonged labor. Prolonged labor can have a number of different causes. One potential cause is if the woman's cervix is not dilating (opening) properly in response to the contractions. This can happen if the cervix is especially stiff or if there is something blocking the cervix from opening, such as a large fibroid. Another potential cause of prolonged labor is if the baby is not in the ideal position for labor to progress.

Question 201:

answer) Option

D)All of the above

When a pregnancy extends beyond 42 weeks, it is considered post-term. While most post-term babies are born healthy, there are some potential complications that can occur.

One complication that can occur is meconium aspiration. Meconium is the baby's first stool, and it is typically green in color. It can be sticky and thick and is typically passed before birth. In some cases, however, meconium can be present in the amniotic fluid. If this happens, there is a risk that the baby could inhale the meconium, which can lead to lung problems.

Another complication that can occur is cord complications. The umbilical cord is the baby's lifeline to the placenta, and it is typically wrapped around the baby's body. In some cases, however, the cord can become wrapped around the baby's neck, which can cause problems with breathing. Additionally, the cord can become knotted, which can cut off the baby's supply of oxygen.

Peripheral nerve injury can occur when the baby is large and presses on the nerves in the mother's pelvis, causing damage.

Question 202:

Answer :

C. Hemorrhage

Explanation: The most common complication post-delivery is hemorrhage, which is the loss of more than 500 ml of blood within the first 24 hours after childbirth. This can occur due to many causes, including uterine atony (lack of contraction of the uterus), lacerations of the birth canal, and retained placental fragments. While most hemorrhages are treatable with IV fluids and blood transfusions, in some cases they can lead to maternal death.

Question 203:

answer) Option
D)All of the above
Explanation) Cell-saver devices are used in surgery to filter and clean a patient's blood. They work by removing blood from the patient and then separating the blood cells from the plasma. The blood cells are then returned to the patient and the plasma is discarded. These devices can be used during surgery to reduce blood loss and allow the patient to receive their own blood back.

Question 204:

.

Answer: D . Uteroplacental insufficiency.
Explanation: Uteroplacental insufficiency is a condition that is rare but very serious that occurs during pregnancy as a result of improper development of the placenta. This condition is also called as placental dysfunction, or uteroplacental vascular insufficiency. This also occurs with low maternal blood pressure which reduces placental blood flow during uterine contractions. Uteroplacental insufficiency may cause hypotension or hypoxemia.

Question 205:

Answer:
A. Clear color of the urine.
Explanation: The color of urine can vary depending on a number of factors, including the person's diet and hydration levels. Clear urine generally indicates that a person is well-hydrated and is not a cause for concern. Other colors of urine, such as yellow or amber, can sometimes indicate dehydration or a urinary tract infection. However, it is important to note that the color of urine can also vary due to things like food coloring or certain medications, so it is not always an accurate indicator of health. Therefore, clear urine should not be reported as a urinary sign, as it is not necessarily indicative of a problem.

Question 206:

Answer :
A)stool form
EXPLANATION: After a woman gives birth, her bowel movements are assessed for a variety of factors. The stool form, or shape, is not typically assessed. Instead, doctors and other medical professionals usually focus on factors such as the frequency of bowel movements, the consistency of the stool, and the presence of blood in the stool.

Stool form can vary greatly from person to person, and even from day to day for the same person. Therefore, it is not considered to be a reliable indicator of anything. The frequency of bowel movements, on the other hand, can give doctors some insight into how well the mother is healing and recovering from childbirth. If a mother is not having regular bowel movements, it could be a sign that she is not getting enough fiber in her diet or that she is constipated. The consistency of the stool can also be informative. If the stool is very hard or very watery, it could be a sign of a problem. Blood in the stool, meanwhile, is always a cause for concern and should be reported to a doctor immediately.

Question 207:

Answer:
A. Low nutritional Status
Explanation: There are a number of physical signs that may be indicative of substance abuse. One such sign is low nutritional status. When someone is abusing drugs or alcohol, they often do not have the proper nutrition that they need to maintain their health. This can lead to a number of problems, including weight loss, fatigue, and weakened immune systems. Another physical sign of substance abuse is changes in appearance. Someone who is abusing drugs or alcohol may have changes in their skin, hair, and nails. They may also have changes in their weight, sleeping habits, and energy levels.

Question 208:

Answer:
A. Hypoplastic left heart syndrome
EXPLANATION: Hypoplastic left heart syndrome is a congenital heart defect where the left side of the heart does not form correctly in the womb. This can lead to a number of complications including heart failure, stroke, and death. Treatment typically involves surgery to correct the defect and may also require medications or other interventions.

Question 209:

Answer:
B.Fundus
EXPLANATION: When a doctor or other medical professional palpates (feels with their hands) a woman's uterus after she has given birth, the highest point they would feel would be the fundus. The fundus is the uppermost part of the uterus, which is located just below the navel. After a baby is born, the fundus is where the placenta was attached. The fundus is also where the uterine muscles contract during labor, which is why it is often very tender to the touch immediately after childbirth. The fundus will gradually shrink back down to its normal size over the course of several weeks.

.

Question 210:

Answer:

C. Wrong billing code.

Explanation: There are a few potential events that could occur which would not be reportable by the patient to the state. One example would be if the patient received the wrong billing code. In this case, the patient would not be expected to know that the code was incorrect, and therefore would not be able to report it.

Question 211:

Answer :

C. Multiparous women

Explanation: It is well established that afterpains are more common in multiparous women. Multiparous women are defined as women who have given birth to two or more children. There are several reasons why afterpains are more common in multiparous women. One reason is that multiparous women have more uterine contractions postpartum than primiparous women. These contractions help the uterus to shrink back to its pre-pregnancy size and are important for preventing postpartum hemorrhage. However, these contractions can also be quite painful. Another reason that afterpains are more common in multiparous women is that they are more likely to have an episiotomy. An episiotomy is a surgical incision made in the perineum (the area between the vagina and the anus) to enlarge the vaginal opening.

Question 212:

Answer:

B.Brown adipose tissue

EXPLANATION: ATP synthesis and oxidative metabolism are two different processes that take place in the body. ATP synthesis is the process of making ATP, while oxidative metabolism is the process of breaking down molecules to release energy. The main difference between these two processes is that ATP synthesis requires oxygen, while oxidative metabolism does not. Brown adipose tissue is a tissue that contains higher levels of mitochondria, which are necessary for ATP synthesis. Brown adipose tissue is found in areas of the body that are more likely to be exposed to cold temperatures, such as the neck and shoulders. When the body is exposed to cold temperatures, the sympathetic nervous system is activated. This causes the release of norepinephrine, which binds to receptors on the surface of brown adipocytes. This triggers a series of events that lead to the release of energy stored in the form of triglycerides. The triglycerides are broken down by enzymes known as lipases. This process releases free fatty acids, which are transported into the mitochondria.

Question 213:
. **answer: Option**

D) It measures fetal metabolic rate.

Explanation: Intrauterine resuscitation is a medical procedure that is used to help improve the oxygenation of a fetus when they are experiencing distress. This can be done through a number of different methods, but the most common is by inserting a catheter into the umbilical cord and infusing oxygenated fluids. This procedure can help to improve the oxygen saturation of the fetus and help to stabilize their heart rate. It can also be used to help assess the fetal condition and determine if there are any other interventions that may be necessary. It is used to treat hypoxia and reverse acidosis.

Question 214:

Answer :
C. It affects the fetal RBCs
Explanation: There are a few ways that parvovirus B19 can affect a pregnant woman and her fetus. The most common, and most serious, complication is fetal anemia. This is caused when the virus destroys the fetus's red blood cells (RBCs). This can lead to serious health problems for the fetus, including heart failure and death. In some cases, the anemia is so severe that the only way to save the fetus is to deliver it early. Another potential complication of parvovirus B19 infection during pregnancy is hydrops fetalis. This is a condition in which the fluid around the fetus builds up to dangerous levels. This can cause the fetus to have heart failure, and can be fatal.

Question 215:

Answer:
D. All of the above
EXPLANATION: When a fetus is exposed to promethazine in the womb, it can show signs of bradycardia, or a slower-than-normal heart rate. This is because promethazine can act as a depressant on the central nervous system, including the heart. Other potential causes of bradycardia in a fetus include exposure to other drugs that depress the central nervous system, such as alcohol or barbiturates, and certain medical conditions that affect the heart or the nervous system, metabolic acidosis and when the fetus is asleep.

Question 216:
correct answer: Option
B) 104 to 108
Explanation In a nonpregnant woman, the normal PaO2 should be 90 to 100. However, in a pregnant woman, the PaO2 should be 104 to 108. The reason for this is that during pregnancy, the blood volume expands and the amount of oxygen carried in the blood also increases. This increase in oxygen helps to ensure that the developing fetus has an adequate supply of oxygen. In addition, the level of hemoglobin in the blood also increases during pregnancy. This increase in hemoglobin helps to bind more oxygen to the blood, making it available to the fetus. So, while the PaO2 should be slightly higher in a pregnant woman compared to a nonpregnant woman, it is still within the normal range.

Question 217:

answer) Option
A) Nipple stimulation causes release of oxytocin, and it cannot be controlled since it is released naturally.

Explanation: Nipple stimulation refers to the act of stimulating the nipples in order to produce a response. The contraction stress test is a test used to evaluate the heart and its ability to pump blood under stress. The test is done by injecting a substance that makes the heart contract and then measuring how well the heart responds. Nipple stimulation as a way to perform the contraction stress test is unreliable because it can cause the release of oxytocin. Oxytocin is a hormone that is released naturally by the body and it cannot be controlled. When oxytocin is released, it can cause the heart to contract and this can interfere with the results of the test.

Question 218:

Answer:
C. Estimated Date of Delivery

EXPLANATION: EDD is an estimate of when a woman will deliver her baby. It is based on the first day of the woman's last menstrual period (LMP) and takes into account the average length of a pregnancy, which is 40 weeks.

EDD can be helpful in planning for the birth but it is not an exact science. In fact, only about 5% of babies are born on their EDD. The majority of babies are born within a week on either side of their EDD.

Question 219:

Answer:
A. It is normal.

Explanation: A neonate, or newborn, is a baby less than four weeks old. It is normal for a neonate to lose some weight in the first few days after delivery. This weight loss is usually due to loss of fluid and is nothing to be concerned about. However, if a neonate loses more than 10% of its birth weight, it is considered excessive and may be a sign of a problem. If Alice has lost half a pound, she has lost less than 10% of her birth weight and so this is not a cause for concern.

Question 220:

Answer:
D.All of the above

EXPLANATION: A uterine rupture is a serious complication that can occur during pregnancy. It occurs when the normal tissue that holds the uterus together tears, leading to the complete or partial separation of the uterus. This can be a life-threatening emergency for both the mother and the baby. If a uterine rupture is suspected, immediate medical attention is required.

There are three primary ways to treat a uterine rupture: laparotomy, cesarean section, and hysterectomy. A laparotomy is a surgical procedure that involves making a large incision in the abdomen in order to access the uterus. During a laparotomy, the surgeon will repair the rupture and then remove the baby via cesarean section. A cesarean section is a surgical procedure in which the baby is delivered through an incision in the mother's abdomen. When the uterus is removed through surgery, it is called a hysterectomy.

. This is typically only done if the rupture is severe and cannot be repaired.

Question 221:

Answer:
A. Uterine atony.
Explanation: Uterine atony is the medical term for a failure of the uterus to contract after childbirth. This can lead to late hemorrhaging, which is bleeding that occurs more than 24 hours after delivery. While hemorrhage is a common complication of childbirth, late hemorrhage is less common, occurring in 1-2% of births uterus is a muscle that contracts to expel the fetus during childbirth. After delivery, the uterus continues to contract to expel the placenta and stop bleeding. When the uterus is unable to effectively contract, it experiences uterine atony. This can lead to excessive bleeding, as the uterine muscles are unable to properly clamp down on the blood vessels.

Question 222:
Answer A) It is normal and it is called acceleration
Explanation: When a physician performs a vaginal examination on a pregnant woman, it is not uncommon for the fetus' heart rate to increase momentarily. This is perfectly normal and is known as acceleration. There are two main reasons why the fetus' heart rate may increase during a vaginal examination. The first is that the physician's hand may briefly come into contact with the fetal heartbeat, which can startle the fetus and cause an increase in heart rate. The second reason is that the procedure may stimulate uterine contraction, which in turn can also lead to an increase in the fetal heart rate.

Question 223:

Answer:A. Thrush(oral candidiasis)
EXPLANATION: During pregnancy, the levels of the hormone progesterone increase, which can lead to vaginal candidiasis. Progesterone levels are highest during the third trimester, which is why thrush is most common in pregnant women during this time. When the membranes that surround the fetus rupture, there is a risk of the fetus becoming infected with the candida fungus. If the thrush is severe, the fetus may develop oral candidiasis, which is a fungal infection of the mouth and throat. Oral candidiasis can lead to a number of complications, including dehydration, difficulty feeding, and even respiratory distress. Fortunately, candidiasis is treatable with antifungal medications. If a woman is in labor and has a ruptured membrane, she will likely be treated with antifungal medication to prevent the spread of the infection to the fetus.

Question 224:

Answer:
D.95%

EXPLANATION: A woman who is 12 weeks into her pregnancy may notice bleeding and experience a miscarriage. On further investigation, the pregnancy may be found to be ectopic This occurs when the embryo implants itself outside of the uterus, usually in the fallopian tube. About 95% of ectopic pregnancies occur in the fallopian tube. There are a few different reasons why an ectopic pregnancy may occur, but the most common cause is a condition called "tubal occlusion." This is when the fallopian tube is blocked, preventing the egg from traveling down to the uterus. Tubal occlusion can be caused by scar tissue from previous injuries or surgery, endometriosis, or infection. Ectopic pregnancies are usually diagnosed with a pelvic exam, ultrasound, or blood test. If the pregnancy is diagnosed early, it can be treated with medication.

Question 225:
answer: Option
A) Doppler ultrasound device
Explanation: A Doppler ultrasound is a device that is used to monitor fetal heart sounds. This device uses sound waves to create an image of the fetus and the heart. The Doppler ultrasound can be used to detect the baby's heartbeat, as well as to listen to the fetal heartbeat. The Doppler ultrasound can also be used to measure the blood flow through the umbilical cord and placenta.

Question 226:

Answer:
A. Ballard.
Explanation The Ballard score is a tool used by doctors to estimate the gestational age of a fetus. The score is based on the physical development of the fetus, and is divided into three zones: Zone A, Zone B, and Zone C. Zone A includes physical characteristics that are present in all fetuses at a certain gestational age. Zone B includes physical characteristics that are present in some fetuses at a certain gestational age. Zone C includes physical characteristics that are present in few fetuses at a certain gestational age. The fetal age is estimated by adding up the points for each physical characteristic that is present in the fetus.

Question 227:

Answer: C. 30% to 60%
EXPLANATION: A hospital nursery should maintain a humidity level of 30% to 60%. The ideal humidity level for a hospital nursery is around 50%. However, a humidity level of 30% to 60% is still considered safe for newborns. Too much humidity can lead to respiratory problems in newborns, so it is important to keep the humidity level in the nursery at a safe level.

Question 228:

Answer: C.Chorioamnionitis (intra-amniotic infection).
Explanation Chorioamnionitis, also known as intra-amniotic infection, is a serious condition that can occur during pregnancy. Symptoms include red, swollen, and inflamed fetal membranes. This condition can lead to preterm labor and delivery, as well as other complications such as infection in the mother and baby. If chorioamnionitis is suspected, it is important to seek medical attention immediately. Treatment typically includes antibiotics, which can help to clear the infection and prevent further complications.

Question 229:

Answer: B. Infants who require a ventilator to be used

Explanation: BPD typically occurs in infants who require the use of a ventilator. This is because BPD is a form of lung injury that can occur when babies are exposed to high levels of oxygen, which is often necessary when they are on a ventilator. BPD can also occur in premature babies, who are also often exposed to high levels of oxygen. In addition, babies with congenital heart defects or other chronic lung conditions are at risk for developing BPD.

Question 230:
answer: **Option**
D)both a and c

Explanation: EFM, or electronic fetal monitoring, is a tool used to assess the well-being of a fetus during labor. It involves attaching sensors to the mother's abdomen to measure the fetal heart rate and contractions. EFM is used to help determine if the fetus is in distress and may need to be delivered urgently. It can also be used to reassure the mother and her caregivers that the fetus is doing well.

Question 231:
answer) Option
A) It is a form of breathing reflex
Explanation: Fetal hiccups are a form of breathing reflex that is often seen in utero. This reflex is thought to help the fetus practice breathing and to also help clear any amniotic fluid that may have accumulated in the lungs. This reflex typically disappears after birth.

Question 232:

Answer:
A. Fluconazole
EXPLANATION: Infections caused by the yeast Candida are known as candidiasis. They can affect different parts of the body, including the vagina, penis, mouth, throat, and skin. Candida infections are usually harmless, but they can cause severe problems in people with weak immune systems. The most common type of candidiasis is vaginal thrush, which affects women of childbearing age. Other types include oral thrush, which affects the mouth, and skin candidiasis, which affects the skin. Oral thrush usually causes white, sore patches in the mouth, throat, or on the tongue. Skin candidiasis often causes a red, itchy rash. Candida infections can be treated with antifungal drugs called azoles. The most common azole drugs are fluconazole (Diflucan) and clotrimaz.

Question 233:

Answer:
B. Fever
Explanation :

While post-dated pregnancy is generally safe for both the mother and the baby, there are some potential complications that can occur. These include:
-The baby growing too large, which can cause complications during delivery
-The placenta becoming detached from the uterine wall
-The development of gestational diabetes
Fever, however, is not a complication that can occur as a result of post-dated pregnancy. This is because fever is caused by an infection, and post-dated pregnancy is not a condition that leads to infection.

Question 234:

Answer:

D.   Delivery of the placenta

EXPLANATION: Losing weight after giving birth is common and nothing to be concerned about. The average new mother loses between 10 and 12 pounds in the first few weeks postpartum. This weight loss is mainly due to the delivery of the placenta and the loss of fluid retention. The placenta is a large organ that attaches to the uterine wall and provides nutrients and oxygen to the developing baby. It weighs between 1 and 2 pounds and is typically delivered within minutes of the baby.

Question 235:

Answer :

C. 1-2 women who contract chicken pox also contract pneumonia

Explanation: Around 1-2 out of every 10 women who contract chickenpox also develop pneumonia. Pneumonia is an infection of the lungs that can be serious, especially for pregnant women. There is a higher risk for pneumonia during pregnancy because the immune system is weakened. Pregnant women who develop pneumonia may need to be hospitalized and may be at risk for premature labor. The best way to prevent chickenpox and pneumonia is to get the chickenpox vaccine. The chickenpox vaccine is safe for pregnant women and is recommended for women who are pregnant and have never had chickenpox.

Question 236:

Answer:

D. Cephalohematoma.

Explanation: A cephalohematoma is a lump that can occur on the skull of a newborn baby. It is caused by blood accumulating below the periosteum, which is a layer of tissue that covers the bone. Cephalohematomas are usually harmless and will resolve on their own over time. However, in rare cases, they can lead to complications such as infection or anemia.

Question 237:
Answer:
C. Erythema Toxicum.

Explanation: Erythema toxicum is a blotchy, red rash that appears in a full-term infant's upper body. It is a benign, self-limited condition that typically resolves within a few days. Erythema toxicum is thought to be caused by the release of histamine and other inflammatory mediators in response to the presence of certain bacteria or other stimuli in the environment. The rash is often seen in newborns who are exposed to certain types of bacteria, such as Staphylococcus aureus, during delivery. The rash typically appears within the first few days of life and typically resolved within a week.

Question 238:

Answer:

A. Hydrocephalus

EXPLANATION: It is a medical condition in which the ventricles, or cavities, of the brain develop an abnormal buildup of cerebrospinal fluid. This excess fluid puts pressure on the brain and can cause a variety of problems, including intellectual disability, seizures, and headaches. Hydrocephalus can be congenital (present at birth) or acquired (developing after birth). Spina bifida is a birth defect in which there is an incomplete closing of the spinal cord and its associated bones (vertebrae). This results in an open lesion, or "gap," in the spinal cord and vertebrae. Spina bifida can cause a variety of problems, including hydrocephalus, motor and sensory impairments, and problems with bowel and bladder function.

Question 239:

Answer:

A. Fontanelles.

EXPLANATION: The fontanelles are the two soft spots on a baby's head. They are usually referred to as the " anterior fontanelle," which is located at the front of the head, and the "posterior fontanelle," which is located at the back of the head. The fontanelles allow the baby's head to collapse during birth and also give the head some flexibility, which is important for a baby's developing brain. The fontanelles begin to close around the age of two and are usually completely fused by the age of eighteen months. However, it is not unusual for the anterior fontanelle to close as early as three months or as late as twelve months. The posterior fontanelle usually closes around six to eight weeks after birth .

Question 240:
Answer:

A. Induction of labor

EXPLANATION: During pregnancy, the levels of oxytocin increase gradually until they peak just before labor begins. When labor begins, the level of oxytocin spikes and causes the uterus to contract. The contractions help the baby to move down the birth canal and be born. In some cases, labor does not begin on its own and medical intervention is necessary. One way to start labor is to administer oxytocin through an IV. The synthetic form of oxytocin is given in small doses and the dose is increased gradually until labor begins. Oxytocin is a safe and effective way to start labor. It has been used for many years and has a very good safety record. There are some side effects of oxytocin, such as nausea, vomiting, and headaches.

Question 241:

Answer:
 C. Head is smaller than the normal circumference
EXPLANATION: The condition of microcephaly occurs when an infant's head is smaller than the normal circumference for their age and sex. This can be due to a number of factors, but in this case, it is likely due to infection with the CMV virus. This virus is a common cause of congenital abnormalities, and microcephaly is one of the more severe manifestations. In addition to the smaller head size, infants with microcephaly often have other neurological problems, such as seizures and mental retardation. There is no specific treatment for microcephaly, but early intervention and supportive care can help improve the child's development and quality of life.

Question 242:

Answer:
 C. Mother is Rh negative and the infant is Rh positive.
Explanation: Rh incompatibility happens when the mother is Rh negative and the infant is Rh positive. This happens because the mother's immune system produces antibodies to the Rh protein, which the infant has inherited from the father. These antibodies attack the Rh protein, causing the blood cells to break down. This can lead to anemia and other serious problems for the infant.

Question 243:
ANSWER:
 D.both b and c
Explanation: When responding to this question, there are a few things to take into account. The first is that a pregnancy is typically considered to be 40 weeks, or 9 months, long. A termination at 6-8 weeks would therefore be very early on in the pregnancy. The second thing to consider is that the organs develop at different rates. For example, the heart develops relatively early on, while the brain and lungs develop later. With that said, if a pregnancy was terminated at 6-8 weeks of gestation, both the heart and the brain would be seen in the fetus. The heart would be beating, and the brain would be beginning to develop. The lungs would not be seen, as they typically develop around week 10-12.

Question 244

Answer:
A.Supplies nutrients to the fetus

EXPLANATION: The placenta is a key organ in the development of a fetus. It is a temporary organ that forms during pregnancy and attaches to the wall of the uterus. The placenta provides nutrients, oxygen, and blood to the growing fetus. It also removes waste products from the fetus. The placenta is connected to the fetus by the umbilical cord. The placenta forms from tissue that grows from the fertilized egg. This tissue attaches to the wall of the uterus and begins to form blood vessels. The placenta grows as the fetus develops. By the end of pregnancy, the placenta is about the size of a dinner plate. The placenta has two main functions. First, it provides nutrients to the fetus. The placenta is rich in iron and essential vitamins. These nutrients are essential for the growth and development of the fetus. Second, the placenta removes waste products from the fetus.

Question 245:

Answer:
D. Neonatal squamous cell test.
EXPLANATION: Neonatal Abstinence Syndrome (NAS) is a set of problems that occur in newborns when they are exposed to drugs while in the womb. The most common drugs that can cause NAS are opioids, such as heroin, but other drugs such as alcohol, barbiturates, and benzodiazepines can also cause the syndrome. The symptoms of NAS can vary from mild to severe and can include tremors, convulsions, and seizures. The severity of the symptoms depends on the type and amount of drug the baby was exposed to, as well as the gestational age of the baby. There is no one test that can diagnose NAS, but the most common method of assessment is the Neonatal squamous cell test. This system uses a set of criteria to score the severity of the baby's symptoms, and is then used to determine the best course of treatment.

Question 246:

Answer:
C. Early deceleration
EXPLANATION: This is considered as early deceleration. Early deceleration is a decrease in fetal heart rate that begins immediately after the start of a uterine contraction and returns to the baseline fetal heart rate after the contraction has ended. It is usually a sign that the baby is tolerating labor well.

Question 247:

Answer:
B. Dilation and curettage (D&C).
EXPLANATION: A molar pregnancy is a pregnancy in which the embryo does not develop, but instead a mass of abnormal tissue grows in the uterus. This condition is also called a hydatidiform mole or gestational trophoblastic disease (GTD). The most common symptom of a molar pregnancy is vaginal bleeding. In some cases, the bleeding may be heavy. Other symptoms may include: - Nausea and vomiting - An enlarged uterus - Excessive thirst - Frequent urination -Passing tissue from the vagina Molar pregnancies are diagnosed using blood tests and ultrasounds. If the pregnancy is suspected to be a molar pregnancy, a dilation, and curettage (D&
C) will be performed. D&C is a surgical procedure in which the cervix is dilated and a curette (a sharp instrument) is used to remove tissue from the uterus. Typically, this treatment is carried out while completely unconscious. D&C is the recommended treatment for molar pregnancies.

Question 248:

 Answer: D.All of the above

EXPLANATION: WRONG The treatment for placenta previa is blood transfusion, hospitalization of the patient, and C-section.

Blood transfusion is necessary to replace the blood loss due to placenta previa. Hospitalization of the patient is required to monitor the patient and to prepare for C-section. C-section is done to deliver the baby and to avoid complications like hemorrhage.

Question 249:

Answer:

C.10 to 12 pounds

EXPLANATION: It is common for new mothers to lose 10 to 12 pounds in the first few weeks after childbirth. This weight loss is mostly due to the loss of water weight and the shedding of the extra blood and fluid that your body no longer needs. Some of the weight loss may also be due to the loss of fat tissue.

Question 250:

Answer:

 C.12 to 48 hours.

EXPLANATION: During pregnancy, the baby is held in place by the uterus, which is a large muscle. The uterus is also supported by ligaments and the pelvic bones. The cervix, which is the lower part of the uterus, is closed off by a mucus plug. This plug protects the baby from infection.

The membranes that surround the baby are called the amniotic sac. The sac is filled with amniotic fluid, which cushions the baby.

The membranes usually rupture 12 to 48 hours before labor begins. When the membranes rupture, the amniotic fluid leaks out. This is called "water breaking."

If labor does not begin within 24 hours after the membranes have ruptured, the doctor may induce labor.

Question 251:

Answer:

A. Method of breathing.

Explanation: There are a lot of things that go into childbirth classes. One of the things that are covered is the method of breathing. This is important because it helps the mother to relax and to focus on the birth. It also helps to keep the pain under control. There are a few different techniques that can be used when it comes to breathing during childbirth.

Question 252:

Answer :

C. 12 weeks or more

Explanation: For some, their period may return as early as 12 weeks postpartum, while for others it may take longer, sometimes even up to a year or more. There are many factors that can affect when the period will return, such as whether you are exclusively breastfeeding or not, how often you are breastfeeding, and your baby's age. If you are exclusively breastfeeding, your period may not return until you wean your baby. This is because when you breastfeed, your body produces the hormone prolactin, which helps to suppress ovulation and prevent your periods from returning. So, the longer you breastfeed, the longer you may have to wait for your period to resume. Additionally, if you are breastfeeding frequently (8-10 times per day), this can also help to delay the return of your periods.

Question 253:

Answer:
 D. Weight

EXPLANATION: A vital sign is used to measure and monitor the health of a patient. It is generally taken before and during medical examinations in order to assess the overall health of a patient and to track any changes in the health of the individual over time. It is important for physicians to have an understanding of a patient's vital signs in order to best diagnose any issues or concerns in the individual.

When it comes to a postpartum woman, there are certain important vital signs that need to be examined during her postpartum period. These are used to monitor her health and progress during her recovery from pregnancy and childbirth. They are used to assess her overall health to ensure she is doing well, and to check for any indicators of complications and other health issues.

Some of the vital signs that are generally taken for a postpartum woman include temperature, pulse rate, respiration rate, blood pressure, and oxygen saturation. Weight is not a vital sign. These are all essential measurements that are taken to assess the overall health of the patient and track any changes in her health.

Question 254

Answer:
A. Sphingomyelin

EXPLANATION: A surfactant is a substance that lowers the surface tension of a liquid, making it easier to spread. In the human body, surfactants are produced by the cells lining the alveoli (air sacs) of the lungs. When a person breathes in, the surfactant coats the alveoli and prevents them from collapsing. A surfactant is first detected in the amniotic fluid at 28 to 32 weeks of pregnancy. It is composed of lipids (fats), proteins, and carbohydrates. The major lipid is sphingomyelin, which makes up 50 to 70 percent of the surfactant. The proteins include surfactant-associated protein A (SP-A) and surfactant-associated protein D (SP-D). The carbohydrates include lactosylceramide and gangliosides.

Question 255:
Answer: A.Fetal movement can be assessed after 28 weeks

EXPLANATION: Fetal movement can easily be detected after 28 weeks. By feel, a healthcare provider can often tell if a baby is alive and kicking. If fetal movement is not observed, it may be a sign of a potential problem and warrant further investigation. In the final weeks of pregnancy, some healthcare providers may use a special stethoscope to listen for the baby's heartbeat. This can be done as early as 24 weeks gestation. If the fetal heartbeat is not detected, it is important to determine if the baby has died or if there is another problem, such as a uterine fibroid, causing the death. Around 28 weeks, most babies are about 10 inches long from head to toe and weigh about 1 1/2 pounds .They can now yawn, hiccup, and make other facial expressions. Just like full-grown adults, they spend much of their time sleeping.

Question 256:

Answer:

B. 30 minutes

   Explanation: When a patient is considered to have Placenta Accreta, it means that the placenta is not delivered within 30 minutes of delivery of the infant. This can be a dangerous situation for both the mother and the baby, as it can lead to hemorrhaging and other complications.   If the placenta is not delivered within 30 minutes of delivery of the baby, the mother may experience hemorrhaging, as the placenta is still attached to the uterus. This can be a dangerous situation for both the mother and the baby, as it can lead to severe blood loss and other complications. In some cases, the placenta may need to be manually removed by a doctor, which can be a risky procedure. Placenta accreta is a potentially life-threatening condition that should be treated by a team of specialists.

Question 257:

Answer:

A. Genetically.

Explanation: When a pregnant woman has genital herpes, it is possible for the virus to be passed to the baby. This can happen during the delivery if the baby comes into contact with the herpes virus in the birth canal. Additionally, if a woman has an active herpes outbreak at the time of labor and delivery, a cesarean section may be necessary to prevent the transmission of the virus to the baby. After the delivery, it is possible for a baby to contract herpes through contact with infected secretions on the mother's breasts. Therefore, it is important for mothers with genital herpes to avoid breastfeeding their infants.

Question 258:

Answer :

C. Empty breasts

Explanation: Mastitis is an inflammation of the breast that is most often caused by an infection. The infection can be bacterial or fungal, and it can occur anywhere in the breast, including the nipple and areola. The symptoms of mastitis include pain, redness, warmth, and swelling in the affected area. The breast may also feel lumpy or hard, and the nipple may be crusty or cracked. Mastitis is most common in women who are breastfeeding, but it can also occur in women who are not pregnant or breastfeeding.

Question 259

Answer :
A. complete

Explanation : Abruptio placenta is when the placenta partially or completely separates from the uterus before delivery. Placental abruption is a serious complication of pregnancy and can occur at any time during pregnancy, but it is most common in the third trimester. Placental abruption can cause heavy bleeding and is a leading cause of maternal and fetal death. There are two types of placental abruption: 1. Partial abruption – this is when the placenta partially separates from the uterus. Partial abruption is the most common type of abruption and is usually not as serious as complete abruption. 2. Complete abruption – this is when the placenta completely separates from the uterus. Complete abruption is a life-threatening emergency and can cause heavy bleeding, shock, and death. In Daisy's case, she has a complete placental abruption. This is a serious complication and can be fatal for both mother and baby.

Question 260:

Answer :
C. Functional residual capacity

Explanation : The amount of air still in the lungs following a typical expiration is known as the functional residual capacity (FRC). It is typically about 2.5 L for an adult. The FRC is the sum of the residual volume (RV) and the expiratory reserve volume (ERV). The FRC is important because it represents the volume of air available for gas exchange during quiet respiration. When the lungs are at FRC, the alveoli are maximally inflated and the airways are open. This minimizes dead space and maximizes the surface area available for gas exchange. One of the key functions of the FRC is to maintain a positive intrapulmonary pressure. This pressure is created by the elastic recoil of the lungs and the surface tension of the alveolar walls. The intrapulmonary pressure is positive because it is greater than the atmospheric pressure.

Question 261:
answer: Option
D)both a and c

Explanation:
Vibroacoustic stimulation (VAS) is a technique used to provide reassurance of fetal well-being during pregnancy. It involves placing a small device over the abdomen of the mother and emitting sounds at a predetermined level. The sound waves vibrate the mother's abdominal tissues, which in turn stimulates the fetus.
VAS is a non-invasive technique that has been shown to be safe and effective in multiple studies. It has been used for over 20 years and is currently approved for use in over 30 countries. VAS is typically used during the second and third trimesters of pregnancy, as it is thought to be most effective during this time.

Question 262:

Answer:
C. Loss of hair.

Explanation: Loss of hair is not seen during the postpartum period. This is because, during pregnancy, the hair follicles are in a resting phase and do not produce new hair. After childbirth, the hair follicles return to their normal growth cycle and new hair begins to grow.

Question 263:

Answer :
 D. B and C

Explanation: After a woman gives birth, it's important for her to take care of her perineum – the area between the vagina and anus. This is especially true if she had an episiotomy, which is a small cut made in the perineum to help the baby come out.

A sitz bath is a great way to clean the perineum and promote healing. It involves sitting in a tub of warm water for 10-15 minutes, multiple times a day. This helps to soothe the area and keeps it clean.

Pericare is another important part of postpartum care. This involves gently cleaning the perineum with a mild soap and water after each urination or bowel movement. This helps to prevent infection and speeds up healing.

Both of these interventions – sitz baths and pericare – are important for women who have delivered vaginally, especially if they had an episiotomy. These simple steps will help to ensure a healthy and speedy recovery.

Question 264:
 answer: Option
 C)Late deceleration

Explanation: A symmetric fall in the heart rate of the fetus following peak uterine contractions is called late deceleration. This occurs when the baby's head is pushed down against the mother's cervix during a contraction. This can cause the baby's heart rate to slow down. Late decelerations are the most common type of deceleration and are usually not a cause for concern. However, if they are severe or occur with other types of decelerations, they may be a sign of a problem.

Question 265
 ANSWER: A) Maternal depression, postpartum depression

explanation: A mother who has delivered a baby may experience a range of different emotions. These can range from elation and happiness to more negative emotions such as anxiety, depression, and even post-traumatic stress disorder. It is not uncommon for mothers to feel overwhelmed and unsupported in the early weeks and months after childbirth. This can lead to feelings of depression, anxiety and isolation. There are a number of different risk factors that can contribute to postpartum depression. These include a history of depression or other mental health issues, a lack of social support, financial stress, Relationship difficulties, sleep deprivation and feelings of guilt or inadequacy. Postpartum depression is the most likely diagnosis for a mother who exhibits signs of depression, mood swings, and a mood disorder. This is a form of clinical depression that can occur in the weeks and months after childbirth. It is thought to be caused by a combination of hormonal changes, psychological factors and social factors.

Question 266:
Answer : C) Bright room

There are several non-pharmacological interventions that can be used to support a newborn with withdrawal symptoms. These include providing a calm and quiet environment, swaddling the baby, providing skin-to-skin contact, and using a pacifier.

Bright light is not typically used as a non-pharmacological intervention for newborns with withdrawal symptoms.

Question 267:

Answer:
A. Occiput posterior presentation.

Explanation: In an occiput posterior presentation, the baby's head is facing down and towards the mother's back. This is the most abnormal presentation during pregnancy because it can cause the baby's head to become trapped during delivery. This can lead to serious complications for both the mother and the baby, including brain damage, spinal cord damage, and even death. This type of presentation is more common in first-time pregnancies and is more likely to occur in women who are carrying twins or who have had a previous cesarean delivery. An occiput posterior presentation can also be caused by a birth defect or an injury to the baby during pregnancy. If an occiput posterior presentation is suspected, the mother will be closely monitored during the remainder of her pregnancy. If the baby's head begins to emerge during delivery, the doctor may attempt to manually turn the head to a more favorable position. In some cases, cesarean delivery may be necessary to avoid complications.

Question 268

Answer:
B. Poor suck reflex.

Explanation When a baby is being monitored for fetal alcohol syndrome, the medical professional must assess for a number of different symptoms and signs. One of the most important signs to look for is a poor suck reflex. This can be indicative of a number of different problems, including brain damage and problems with muscles or nerves. The poor suck reflex is often one of the first signs of fetal alcohol syndrome. It can be difficult to assess, as it can be subtle. Often, the medical professional will ask the mother to observe the baby while they are feeding. If the baby has a poor suck reflex, it may have trouble latching on to the nipple, or may not be able to suck effectively. This can lead to weight loss or failure to thrive. In addition to the poor suck reflex, the medical professional will also assess for other signs of fetal alcohol syndrome. These can include facial abnormalities, growth retardation, and problems with the central nervous system. If any of these signs are present, the diagnosis of fetal alcohol syndrome is likely.

Question 269:
Answer:
D. Often hard to obtain a required tracing.

Explanation: Often hard to obtain a required tracing. A fetus's welfare is evaluated using the NST (Non-Stress Test). It is often used when there are concerns about the growth or development of the fetus, or when the mother has a medical condition that may affect the fetus. The test involves attaching sensors to the mother's abdomen, which measure the fetal heart rate and the mother's contractions. The test is usually done in two stages, with the first stage lasting around 20 minutes and the second stage lasting around 40 minutes. During the test, the mother is usually asked to walk on a treadmill or ride a stationary bike. The fetal heart rate is monitored during the test and should increase when the mother exerts herself. The test is considered to be positive if the fetal heart rate increases by at least 15 beats per minute for at least 15 seconds. A disadvantage of the NST is that it can often be hard to obtain a required tracing. This may be due to the mother's movements during the test, or the position of the fetus.

Question 270:
Answer:
A.150-400.

Explanation: When a woman is pregnant, her blood volume increases by approximately 50%. This increase in blood volume leads to an increase in the number of circulating red blood cells, white blood cells, and platelets. The bone marrow, where these blood cells are produced, ramps up production in response to the increased demand. Maternal platelet count is a measure of the number of platelets in a pregnant woman's blood. Platelets are small blood cells that help the blood to clot. A platelet count of 150 to 400 is considered normal.

Question 271:

answer) Option
B)1-3%

Explanation) Polyadramnios is a condition that occurs during pregnancy in which there is an excessive amount of amniotic fluid surrounding the fetus. This condition can occur for a variety of reasons, including twins or triplets, pregnancy-induced hypertension, diabetes, and certain types of birth defects. Polyadramnios can also occur in cases where the mother has had a previous stillbirth or miscarriage. While the exact prevalence of polyadramnios is unknown, it is estimated to occur in 1-3% of all pregnancies. Polyadramnios can cause a number of complications for both the mother and the baby.

Question 272

Answer:
C.Zavanelli maneuver.

Explanation A Zavanelli maneuver is a medical procedure in which the head of the fetus is pushed back into the birth canal. This is typically done during a cesarean or C-section procedure. The maneuver is named after Giuseppe Zavanelli, who first described it in a medical journal in 1977. The Zavanelli maneuver is typically used when the fetus is in a breech position (bottom first) and the head cannot be delivered vaginally. The maneuver is also sometimes used when the umbilical cord is prolapsed (hanging down into the birth canal). The Zavanelli maneuver is considered a last resort because it carries a high risk of fetal mortality. In some cases, the maneuver can result in the fetus becoming stuck in the birth canal. If this happens, an emergency cesarean or C-section must be performed. While the Zavanelli maneuver is considered a high-risk procedure, it may be the only option if a vaginal delivery is not possible.

Question 273

Answer:

A. Incompetent cervix.

Explanation: Cervical cerclage is performed when the cervix is determined to be incompetent, or unable to support a pregnancy. This can be due to a number of factors, including a previous history of miscarriage or preterm labor. Incompetent cervix is also referred to as cervical insufficiency. There are two types of cervical cerclage: transcervical and transabdominal. Transcervical cerclage is performed through the vagina and cervix, while transabdominal cerclage is performed through the abdomen. The type of cerclage performed will depend on the individual case and the severity of the incompetence. Cervical cerclage is a safe and effective way to prevent miscarriage and preterm labor in women with an incompetent cervix. It is important to note that not all women with an incompetent cervix will require a cerclage. In some cases, the cervix may be strengthened enough to support a pregnancy without the need for surgery.

Question 274:

Answer:

A.   Birth assisting instruments

EXPLANATION: During labor, broken bones can occur for a variety of reasons. The most common cause is from the baby's head pressing on the mother's pelvic bones. This can happen if the baby is too large to fit through the mother's pelvis, if the baby is in the wrong position, or if the mother has a small pelvis. Other causes of broken bones during labor include forceps or vacuum extraction, breech birth, and twins or more. Broken bones during labor are usually not serious and heal within a few weeks.

Question 275:
answer: Option
C)both a and b
Explanation: A cord blood gas analysis is performed when there is a risk of neonatal encephalopathy or the mother has a thyroid disorder. This test measures the amount of oxygen and carbon dioxide in the blood, as well as the pH level. This information is used to determine how well the baby's lungs are functioning and whether the mother's thyroid disorder is having any effect on the baby's oxygen levels.

Question 276

Answer:

B. Preterm birth.

Explanation: Placenta previa is a condition that can occur during pregnancy in which the placenta partially or completely covers the cervix. This can cause bleeding during pregnancy and can be dangerous for both the mother and the baby. Placenta previa can also cause premature birth.

Question 277

answer: Option

B) Caudal agenesis

Explanation: A newborn born to a diabetic mother shows agenesis of the lumbar spine, sacrum and coccyx. There is a hypoplasia of the lower extremities. The most probable diagnosis in this case is caudal agenesis. Caudal agenesis is a rare congenital disorder characterized by the partial or complete absence of the bones of the lower spine (lumbar spine, sacrum, and coccyx). This results in shortened and deformed lower limbs. The condition is caused by a problem with the development of the lower spinal cord during fetal development. The majority of cases of caudal agenesis are diagnosed at birth. The characteristic findings on physical examination are shortened and deformed lower limbs, with the degree of deformity depending on the severity of the condition.

Question 278

Answer: C.1-3 hours.

EXPLANATION: The average length of labor is around twelve hours for a first-time mother. However, for a woman who has already had a baby, labor may only last around six hours. In some cases, labor can be much shorter - this is known as precipitous labor. Precipitous labor is defined as labor that lasts less than three hours from the onset of contractions to the delivery of the baby. There are a number of possible explanations for why precipitous labor may occur. One possibility is that the woman's pelvic floor muscles are particularly strong and efficient at pushing the baby out. Another possibility is that the baby is in a favorable position for delivery, known as an occiput anterior position. This position allows the baby to descend down the birth canal more quickly.

Question 279:

answer: D. Chorioangioma

EXPLANATION:A chorioangioma is a benign tumor that develops on the placenta. These tumors are usually asymptomatic and do not cause any harm to the mother or baby. However, in rare cases, they can grow large enough to cause placental insufficiency or preterm labor. Chorioangiomas are made up of abnormal blood vessels. Chorioangiomas usually do not grow any larger than 5 cm in diameter.

Question 280

Answer:

D. 3rd or immediately after delivery.

Explanation: Acute fatty liver of pregnancy (AFLP) is a rare but potentially fatal complication that can occur during the last few months of pregnancy. The exact cause is unknown, but it is thought to be related to a build-up of fat in the liver. Failure and liver damage may result from this. AFLP usually occurs in the third trimester of pregnancy, but it can also occur in the first two weeks after delivery. The symptoms of AFLP can vary from mild to severe, and can include: - Nausea and vomiting - Jaundice (yellowing of the skin and eyes) - Enlarged liver - Abdominal pain - Fatigue .

Question 281:
Answer :

A. condensation

Explanation: When we think of the ways we lose heat, we typically think of convection, radiation, and evaporation. Condensation is not a mechanism of heat loss. Condensation is the process by which a gas turns into a liquid. This can happen when a gas is cooled below its dew point, or when it comes into contact with a surface that is cooler than the gas.

Question 282:
Answer:

A. Involution.

Explanation: The process of involution is the return of the uterus to its non-pregnant state from its pregnant state. This is a physiological process that occurs naturally after the delivery of a baby. The process of involution begins immediately after the delivery of the baby and the placenta and can take up to 6 weeks to complete. The uterus must undergo a series of changes in order to return to its non-pregnant state. The first change is the involution of the placental site. The placenta is attached to the uterine wall during pregnancy and provides nutrients and oxygen to the developing baby. The placenta leaves the body after delivery because it is no longer required. The expulsion of the placenta trigger's the start of involution. The uterine muscles must also contract in order to return to their pre-pregnancy state. These contractions help the uterus to expel the remaining tissue and blood from the pregnancy. The contractions also help the cervix to close and return to its normal size.

Question 283:
answer: Option C: hypotension due to epidural

Explanation: It is most likely that the pregnant woman is experiencing hypotension due to the epidural. This is a condition in which the blood pressure becomes too low, and can cause a variety of symptoms like those listed. Some other potential causes of the symptoms could be an allergic reaction to the medication used in the epidural, or a reaction to the anesthetic itself. However, hypotension is the most likely cause, and can be treated by increasing the woman's fluid intake and lying her down on her left side.

Question 284:

Answer :

C. check latching or baby's positioning

Explanation : A bad latch can cause sore nipples. Observe these indications of a quality latch: The baby's chin touches the breast. The baby's lips are turned out (flanged). You can see more of the areola above the baby's top lip than below the bottom lip. The baby's tongue is cupped under the breast. You can hear quiet sucking sounds, not clicking noises. The way the baby is positioned can also cause sore nipples.

Question 285:
Answer :

B. Abruptio placenta

Explanation: Placental abruption, or abruptio placentae, is a serious pregnancy complication in which the placenta partially or completely separates from the uterine wall before delivery. Placental abruption can occur at any point during pregnancy, but it is most common during the third trimester. Placental abruption is a medical emergency and can be life-threatening for both the mother and the baby. If the abruption is severe, it can cause the baby to be born prematurely or to suffer from a lack of oxygen (asphyxia). Placental abruption can also cause heavy bleeding (hemorrhage) in the mother, which can be life-threatening.

Question 286

Answer: A. Subcapsular hematoma

EXPLANATION: A subcapsular hematoma is a medical emergency that can potentially lead to liver failure. This occurs when there is bleeding underneath the liver capsule, which is the membrane that encloses and protects the liver. This can cause the liver to become enlarged and rupture. Symptoms of a subcapsular hematoma may include abdominal pain, jaundice, and fever. If the hematoma is large, it can cause the liver to fail. This is a surgical emergency that needs to be handled right away. Treatment for a subcapsular hematoma includes surgery to remove the hematoma and repair any damage to the liver.

Question 287:
Answer:

A. Ectoderm.

Explanation: Germ cells are cells that give rise to gametes, which are the cells that fuse together during sexual reproduction to form a zygote. The zygote then goes on to develop into an embryo. Germ cells can be found in both sexes, and they originate from different parts of the body in males and females. In males, germ cells originate in the testes, and in females, they originate in the ovaries. The outer layer of germ cells is called the ectoderm. The ectoderm gives rise to the skin, nails, hair, and nervous system. It also helps to form certain glands, such as the sweat glands and the oil glands. The ectoderm is the first layer of cells to develop in the embryo, and it is also the layer of cells that covers the surface of the embryo.

Question 288:

answer) Option
D)Both a and b

Explanation) A biophysical score is a tool used to assess the health and viability of a fetus. The score is based on a number of factors, including the fetus's heart rate, breathing, muscle tone, and amniotic fluid levels. A high score indicates a healthy fetus, while a low score indicates an unhealthy fetus. The biophysical score is used to assess the fetus's well-being and is an important tool for doctors in making decisions about whether or not to intervene in a pregnancy. A high score indicates that the fetus is healthy and is likely to survive outside the womb, while a low score indicates that the fetus is unhealthy and is at risk for complications or death. There are a number of different biophysical scores, but the most common is the Fetal Activity Level (FAL) score. The FAL score is based on the fetus's heart rate, breathing, and muscle tone. A score of 8 or higher indicates a healthy fetus, while a score of 7 or lower indicates an unhealthy fetus.

Question 289:

Answer: C . Do Caesarean section
Explanation: In cases where the baby is breech, meaning that the baby is positioned to come out feet-first rather than head-first, interventions are usually necessary in order to ensure a safe delivery. The most common intervention is a Caesarean section, which is a surgical procedure in which the baby is delivered through an incision in the mother's abdomen. In some cases, an external cephalic version (ECV) may be attempted, which is a procedure in which the doctor manually tries to manipulate the baby into a head-first position. However, this is only successful about half of the time, and if it is unsuccessful, a Caesarean section will likely be necessary.

Question 290:
answer: Option
B)Gonorrhea
Explanation: The patient is most likely suffering from gonorrhea, a sexually transmitted infection (STI) caused by the bacteria Neisseria gonorrhoeae. The infection is usually transmitted through sexual contact, including vaginal, anal, and oral sex. During childbirth, a mother may also transmit gonorrhea to the unborn child. Symptoms of gonorrhea include watery, creamy or greenish vaginal discharge, pain or burning while urinating, pain during penetrative vaginal intercourse, and heavier periods or spotting. In some cases, gonorrhea can cause no symptoms at all. If left untreated, gonorrhea can lead to serious health complications, including pelvic inflammatory disease, infertility, and an increased risk of HIV infection. Treatment for gonorrhea usually involves a course of antibiotics.

Question 291:

Answer:
D. Implementation.
Explanation The Gynecology Nurses' Association (GNA) is a professional organization for nurses who specialize in the care of women with gynecologic disorders. The GNA's Code of Ethics for Gynecologic Nurses includes six ethical principles that guide the practice of gynecologic nursing: beneficence, nonmaleficence, autonomy, justice, fidelity, and veracity. Implementation is not included as one of the six ethical principles in the GNA's Code of Ethics for Gynecologic Nurses.

Question 292

Answer:

A. nifedipine

Explanation A vulval hematoma is a pooling of blood in the vulva, the external genitalia of females. It is a relatively rare condition, but can cause significant pain and swelling. Treatment typically involves aggressive conservative measures, such as bed rest, ice packs, and pain medication. If these fail to resolve the hematoma, then surgery may be necessary to remove the blood and relieve the pressure. Nifedipine is a medication that is used to treat high blood pressure and angina. It is not used to treat vulval hematomas.

Question 293

answer: Option

D)Both a and c

Explanation: Ultrasound scanning is performed both transvaginally and abdominally in pregnant women. Transvaginal ultrasound is most often used during early pregnancy, before the fetal heartbeat can be seen on an abdominal ultrasound, and is also used to evaluate the uterus and ovaries in women of childbearing age who are not pregnant. Abdominal ultrasound may be used during any stage of pregnancy. It is most commonly used to assess the baby's growth and to screen for birth defects after the fetal heart beat has been seen.

Question 294

Answer:

D. Vaginal discharge that is severe

EXPLANATION: A vulval hematoma is a pooling of blood that occurs outside of blood vessels. This can happen due to trauma, such as from childbirth, surgery, or an injury. The blood becomes trapped and forms a mass. Symptoms of a vulval hematoma can vary depending on the size and location of the mass. They may include vulvar pain, swelling, bruising, and change in the appearance of the vulva. Vaginal discharge that is severe is not a symptom of a vulval hematoma.

Question 295:

Answer: C. 4th stage

EXPLANATION: In the fourth stage of labor, the baby is born and the placenta is delivered. After the baby is born, the umbilical cord is clamped and cut, and the baby is weighed and measured. The baby is then placed on the mother's chest for skin-to-skin contact. The mother and baby are then checked for any injuries or bleeding. The perineum (area between the vagina and anus) is also checked for any tears or damage. After the birth, the mother will continue to bleed for six to eight weeks postpartum. During this time, she will need to use pads to absorb the blood flow. The mother will also experience afterpains as the uterus contracts back to its pre-pregnancy size. These contractions can be quite painful and may last for several hours or days. The mother may also have a bloody discharge for several weeks as the uterus expels the remains of the placenta.

Question 296:

Answer:

A. 25%.

Explanation: The head makes up a quarter of an infant's body immediately after birth. This is because the head is the largest part of the body and the body is mostly water. The water makes up approximately 80% of the total body weight. The head accounts for about 10% of the body's weight. The remaining body weight is made up of the trunk, arms, and legs. The head-to-body ratio is highest at birth and gradually decreases over the first year of life. By one year of age, the head makes up about one-seventh of the total body weight. The head-to-body ratio is higher in males than females and in whites than in blacks. The size of the head also changes in the first year of life. The head circumference decreases from an average of 35 cm at birth to 32 cm at one year of age. The head size relative to the body size also decreases over the first year.

Question 297:

Answer: D. All of the above

Exlplanation:

During pregnancy, the uterus expands to accommodate the growing fetus. The uterus is a muscular organ, and the extra weight and size put stress on the muscles and ligaments that support it. After childbirth, the uterus must contract back down to its normal size and shape. The process of involution begins immediately after the baby is born and the placenta is delivered.

The first stage of involution, known as expulsion, occurs as the uterus contracts to expel the placenta and any remaining tissue. The second stage, known as retraction, occurs as the uterus shrinks back down to its normal size. The final stage, known as restitution, occurs as the uterine tissue is reabsorbed and the cervix and vagina return to their prepregnant state.

Involution is a natural process that happens without intervention. However, certain factors can affect the process. These include the mother's age, the number of previous pregnancies, the baby's weight, and the use of any medications or medical interventions during labor and delivery.

Question 298:

Answer:

   A. redness and swelling at the site

Explanation:

Infections after a c section are not uncommon. The most common symptom of an infection is a fever, but other symptoms may include redness, swelling, or drainage from the incision site. A few more symptoms include:

- The temperature is above 100.4°F (38°C)
- Feelings of chills
- Incision discharge that smells foul
- Incisions that are red, swollen, or warm
- Incision-related pain
- A feeling of nausea

Question 299:

Answer:

B)7-9 weeks
It is common for periods to take a few weeks to return after pregnancy and childbirth. However, some women may experience anovulation, which is when the ovaries do not release an egg. This can cause irregularities in the menstrual cycle and may cause periods to become less frequent or even stop altogether.

After you give birth, the body needs time to recover and heal. This process is different for everyone, but generally speaking, it takes anywhere from 7 to 9 weeks for periods to return after pregnancy.

During this time, the body is going through a lot of changes as it adjusts to life post-pregnancy. Hormone levels are also shifting, which can impact the menstrual cycle. Breastfeeding can further delay the return of periods.

Question 300:
Answer: A. Erythromycin

In newborns, Neisseria gonorrhea can cause a range of serious health problems including pneumonia, meningitis, and sepsis. Newborns are particularly vulnerable to these infections because their immune systems are not yet fully developed. Treatment of Neisseria gonorrhea in newborns is typically with antibiotics. Erythromycin is one such antibiotic, and it is typically used to treat a wide range of other bacterial infections in newborns, as well.

Thank you for purchasing this book!

I know you could have picked any number of books to read, but you picked this book and for that I am extremely grateful.

What Do You Think of this RNC-OB Exam Study Guide?

I hope that this book added value and quality to your life and helped you in your Inpatient Obstetric Exam preparation. If you liked this book and found some benefit in reading this, I'd like to hear from you and hope that you could take some time to post a review on Amazon. Your feedback and support will help me to greatly improve my writing for future projects and make this book even better.

Your review is very important to me as it helps me morally. Hope this book helped you in some way to crack the exam.

Warm Regards,
Sandra H. White